Diagnostic Imaging of Coronary Artery Disease

Diagnostic Imaging of Coronary Artery Disease

Kusai S. Aziz, MD, FACC

Nuclear Cardiologist and Interventional Cardiologist
Visalia Cardiovascular and Medical Center
Visalia, California

George S. Abela, MSc, MD, MBA

Professor and Chief
Division of Cardiology
Department of Medicine
Michigan State University
East Lansing, Michigan

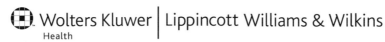

Wolters Kluwer Health

Lippincott Williams & Wilkins

Philadelphia • Baltimore • New York • London
Buenos Aires • Hong Kong • Sydney • Tokyo

Acquisitions Editor: Frances DeStefano
Managing Editor: Leanne McMillan
Marketing Manager: Kimberly Schonberger
Designer: Stephen Druding
Compositor: International Typesetting and Composition

Library of Congress Cataloging-in-Publication Data

Aziz, Kusai.
   Diagnostic imaging of coronary artery disease / Kusai Aziz, George S.
Abela.
      p. ; cm.
   Includes bibliographical references.
   ISBN-13: 978-0-7817-6602-9
   ISBN-10: 0-7817-6602-8
   1. Coronary heart disease—Imaging.   I. Abela, George S.   II. Title.
   [DNLM: 1. Coronary Artery Disease—diagnosis.   2. Diagnostic
Imaging—methods.   WG 300 A995d 2009]
   RC685.C6A95 2009
   616.1'230754—dc22
                                          2008030051

Care has been taken to confirm the accuracy of the information present and to describe generally accepted
practices. However, the authors, editors, and publisher are not responsible for errors or omissions or for any
consequences from application of the information in this book and make no warranty, expressed or implied,
with respect to the currency, completeness, or accuracy of the contents of the publication. Application of this
information in a particular situation remains the professional responsibility of the practitioner; the clinical
treatments described and recommended may not be considered absolute and universal recommendations.

The authors, editors, and publisher have exerted every effort to ensure that drug selection and dosage set
forth in this text are in accordance with the current recommendations and practice at the time of publication.
However, in view of ongoing research, changes in government regulations, and the constant flow of information relating to drug therapy and drug reactions, the reader is urged to check the package insert for each drug
for any change in indications and dosage and for added warnings and precautions. This is particularly important when the recommended agent is a new or infrequently employed drug.

Some drugs and medical devices presented in this publication have Food and Drug Administration (FDA)
clearance for limited use in restricted research settings. It is the responsibility of the health care provider to
ascertain the FDA status of each drug or device planned for use in their clinical practice.

To purchase additional copies of this book, call our customer service department at **(800) 638-3030** or fax
orders to **(301) 223-2320**. International customers should call **(301) 223-2300**.

Visit Lippincott Williams & Wilkins on the Internet: http://www.lww.com. Lippincott Williams & Wilkins
customer service representatives are available from 8:30 am to 6:00 pm, EST.

Cover Image: The Royal Collection © 2008 Her Majesty Queen Elizabeth II.

To my wonderful wife and children, kind parents,
and all my teachers and mentors, I dedicate this work.

Kusai Aziz

To my three boys, Oliver, Andrew and Scott
with pride and joy

George Abela

George S. Abela, MD, MSc, FACC
Division of Cardiology
Department of Medicine
Michigan State University
East Lansing, Michigan

Kim Arellano-Villarreal, MD
Department of Diagnostic Radiology
OSF Saint Francis Medical Center
Department of Radiology
University of Illinois College
   of Medicine at Peoria
Peoria, Illinois

Kusai S. Aziz, MD, FACC
Visalia Cardiovascular and Medical Center
Visalia, California

Kevin L. Berger, MD
Department of Radiology
Michigan State University
East Lansing, Michigan

Kavitha M. Chinnaiyan, MD
Division of Cardiology
William Beaumont Hospital
Royal Oak, Michigan

Ralph E. Gentry, RT, R, MR, CT
Supervisor
Department of Heart and Vascular Disease
William Beaumont Hospital
Royal Oak, Michigan

Henry Gewirtz, MD
Department of Nuclear Cardiology
Massachusetts General Hospital
Cardiac Unit Associates
Boston, Massachusetts

Laxmi S. Mehta, MD
Department of Clinical Internal Medicine
Women's Cardiovascular Health Clinic
Ohio State University Medical Center
Columbus, Ohio

Raymond Q. Migrino, MD, FACC
Cardiovascular Division
Medical College of Wisconsin
Milwaukee, Wisconsin

Gilbert L. Raff, MD
Medical Director
Advanced Cardiovascular Imaging
William Beaumont Hospital
Royal Oak, Michigan

Jack Rubinstein, MD
Clinical Instructor of Medicine
Division of Cardiology
Michigan State University
East Lansing, Michigan

Ibrahim Shah, MD
Assistant Professor of Medicine
Division of Cardiology
Michigan State University
East Lansing, Michigan

Coronary artery disease is the greatest cause of mortality in the United States, and the increasing global incidence is expected to make it the number-one killer worldwide by 2020. Recently the noninvasive detection of coronary artery disease has advanced tremendously in many fields, including nuclear cardiology (both single photon emission tomography and positron emission tomography), computed tomography angiography, and magnetic resonance imaging. Much research is also ongoing in the area of plaque characterization and inflammatory markers. In this book we provide a basic idea about these modalities. Because of time constraints facing clinicians, we tried to explain basic physics concepts in the simplest and clearest manner using examples and hand-drawn figures.

In the CD portion of this book, we provide numerous real-life cases and clinical scenarios to enhance the understanding of basic concepts and interpretation of cardiac single photon emission tomography and computed tomography angiography.

Our work is not intended to be an exhaustive analysis of these imaging modalities; rather, it provides a unique approach to the basic concepts and must-know facts of these modalities. This is especially useful as a rapid entry-level tool for those who are interested in risk stratification of coronary artery disease. The reader can use the information provided as a basis to achieve understanding of basic concepts that can then be further developed by more subspecialized exposure to the field. Also, we include practical tips regarding the establishment of an office-based nuclear cardiology practice.

Finally, we believe that the information and concepts contained in this book can be helpful in preparation for the certifying exam of the Board of Nuclear Cardiology.

CONTENTS

Diagnostic Imaging of Coronary Artery Disease

CHAPTER 1

Kusai S. Aziz

Basic Physics of Single Photon Emission Computed Tomography Physics

This chapter does not deal with the details of nuclear physics, but rather emphasizes basic must-know concepts of nuclear physics that are needed in the practice of nuclear cardiology. Many of these concepts tend to be the subject of board exam questions because of their importance.

Definitions and Basic Principles

1. Basic atomic structure: each atom is composed of a nucleus that contains protons and neutrons, and shells that contain electrons (Figure 1.1).
2. Elements are expressed in a standard fashion to reflect nuclear characteristics (Figure 1.2).
3. The unit of energy is electron volts (eV), defined as the energy or acceleration of an electron obtained by applying electric potential of one volt.
4. Different electromagnetic forces have different levels of energy that increase in an incremental manner: radio waves < TV waves < radar waves < infrared light < visible light < ultraviolet rays < X rays < gamma rays.
5. The frequency and photon energy of any electromagnetic force is inversely related to its wavelength.
6. When an electron moves from an outer shell (higher energy) to an inner shell (lower energy), the excess energy is emitted as a characteristic X-ray or as an Auger electron, which is another electron emitted from an outer shell (Figure 1.3). The probability of X-ray emission versus Auger electron is directly related to the atomic number.
7. Energy and mass are interchangeable: Energy = mass × c (constant, velocity of light).
8. Isotopes have the same number of protons (atomic number, Z); isotones have the same neutron number, N; and isobars have the same mass number, A. Isomers are nuclides of the same element with one of them being in a metastable (unstable) state, e.g., Tc-99m (^{99m}Tc) and ^{99}Tc are isomers. The metastable isomer tends to decay to the stable form by emitting radiation.
9. Radioactive decay: a spontaneous nuclear process in which an unstable nucleus transforms to more stable forms by emitting particles or photons. The original nucleus is called "parent" and the new nucleus is called "daughter," which itself can be a parent and decay further to another "daughter" nucleus. There are different types of decay, as illustrated in Figure 1.4.
10. Units of radioactivity:

    Becquerel (Bq) = 1 disintegration/sec
    Curie (Ci) = 3.7×10^{10} Bq

    The Bq is an SI unit; most medical applications still use the old system (Ci).

FIGURE 1.1 Basic atomic structure.

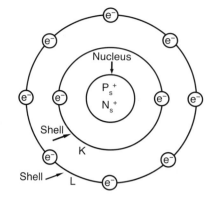

P+ : Proton (positively charged)
N° : Neutron (neutral or no charge)
e− : Electron (negative charge)
Nucleus
Ps+
Ns+
e−
Shell
K
Shell
L

FIGURE 1.2 Expression of elements.

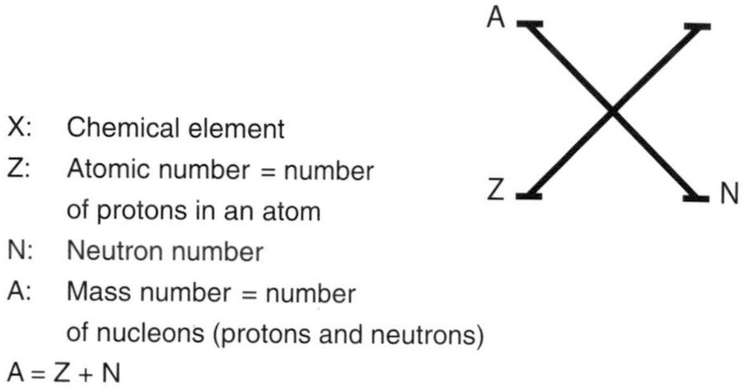

X: Chemical element
Z: Atomic number = number of protons in an atom
N: Neutron number
A: Mass number = number of nucleons (protons and neutrons)
A = Z + N
A
Z
N

e−
Nucleus
either
or
Auger electron
x-ray

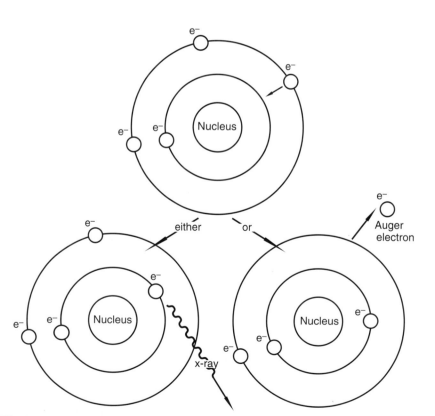

FIGURE 1.3 X-ray or Auger electron emission.

Alpha decay:

$$^A_Z\chi \longrightarrow \, ^{A-4}_{(Z-2)}Y + \, ^4_2He \; (\alpha \, particle)$$

Beta decay (β^-):

$$^A_Z\chi \longrightarrow \, ^{A-1}_{Z+1}Y + e^- + \nu$$

$$n^0 \longrightarrow p^+ + e^- + \nu$$

e^- = electron = Beta particle

ν = neutrino, a particle without mass or charge

Positron emission (β^+):

$$^A_Z\chi = \, ^A_{Z-1}Y + e^+ + \nu$$

$$p^+ \longrightarrow n + e^+ + \nu$$

e^+ = positron = β^+

$e^+ + e^- \; \dfrac{Annihilation}{Reaction}$ 2 photons at 180° of each other. Each one has the energy of a 511 mega electron volt

Electron capture:

$$p^+ + e^- \longrightarrow n^0 + \nu$$

Proton captures electron and converts to neutron followed by emission of x-ray or Auger electron.

Gamma decay (isomeric transmission):

excited nucleus $\longrightarrow$ stable nucleus + γ-ray

FIGURE 1.4 Types of radioactive decay.

11. Physical half-life: the time required for a specific amount of radionuclide or activity to decay to half its original amount. Biological half-life is the time required for the chemical portion of radionuclide to decrease to half its original amount in biological systems, which includes metabolism and excretion. Effective half-life is the time required for the radioactive material to decrease to half its original quantity and this depends on both physical and biological factors.

12. Interaction of energy with matter: when photons or charged particles pass through matter they get absorbed and attenuated. The interaction depends on many factors, including the mass and charge of the particles and the type and thickness of the matter. There are three basic mechanisms of interactions. These include photoelectric effects, Compton effects, and pair production. These mechanisms are illustrated in Figure 1.5.

13. Radiation doses: radiation absorbed dose (rad) is defined as 100 ergs of absorbed energy per gram of substance. The new SI unit gray (Gy) is equivalent to 100 rad. The biological equivalent dose is calculated by multiplying the absorbed dose by a weighing factor, which is 1 in humans. Therefore, the amount of absorbed dose and equivalent doses are the same but the units are different. The equivalent dose is measured in rem (rad equivalent) and sievert (Sv) in international units (Gy equivalent). Sv = 100 rem.

FIGURE 1.5   Mechanisms of energy and matter interaction.

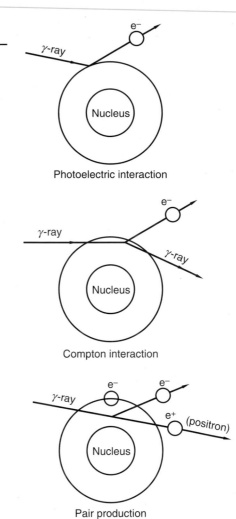

Photoelectric interaction

Compton interaction

Pair production

14. Radionuclide production: radionuclides can be produced by nuclear reactors or accelerators (cyclotrons), or by using generators to produce short-living isotopes. The principle of a generator is that a long-lived radionuclide (parent) decays and is in equilibrium with a daughter nuclide of short half-life. It is the daughter nuclide that is used a tracer. There are two important generators in the field of nuclear cardiology: Tc-99m (SPECT agent) and Rb-82 (PET agent) generators. Four half-lives of the daughter tracer are needed to achieve equilibrium, if parent T/2 daughter T/2 it is called transient equilibrium (e.g., Mo99-Tc99), if parent T/2 daughter T/2 it is called secular equilibrium (e.g., Sr82-Tc99). An outline of the Tc-99m generator is illustrated in Figure 1.6.

Nuclear Tracers and Their Characteristics (Figure 1.7)

Thallium-201 (Tl-201)
- Elemental substance (like K).
- Cyclotron produced.
- Maximum myocardial uptake at 5 minutes.
- Redistributes; therefore, used as viability agent.

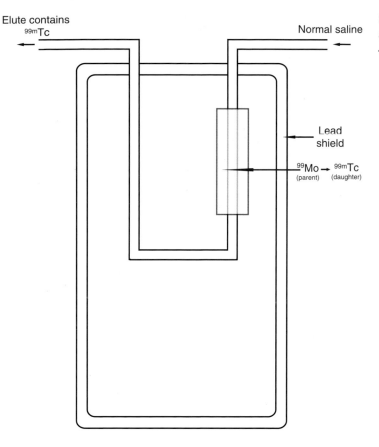

Elute contains
^{99m}Tc

Normal saline

FIGURE 1.6 Basic principles of a ^{99m}Tc generator.

Lead
shield

^{99}Mo → ^{99m}Tc
(parent)   (daughter)

- Imaging should start within 5–10 minutes.
- Increased lung activity suggests ischemia.
- Low cost.
- Good high flow correlation.
- Drawbacks: Long half-life (73 hours) limits dose (4 mCi), low photon energy (80 keV) gives low quality scans, longer acquisition time.
- Most of the radioactivity produced by Thallium is X-ray with energy level of 78 keV; therefore, the nuclear camera acquisition window should be set around that energy level.

Technetium 99-m Sestamibi (Cardiolite®)
- The tracer is attached to isonitrile.
- Relatively short half-life (6 hours), which allows higher dose.
- Tc-99m is generator produced.
- The sestamibi is kit produced.
- Does not redistribute.
- Drawbacks: Considerable hepatobiliary uptake; therefore, should wait before image acquisition. Limited high flow correlation.
- Note: Sestamibi can also be used in the diagnosis of cancer.

Technetium 99-m Testrofosmin (Myoview®)
- Diphosphine (liphophilic agent)
- Rapid hepatobiliary clearance, which allows shorter protocols
- Drawback: Poor high flow correlation (less than sestamibi)

FIGURE 1.7 The relationship between apparent and real myocardial flow for different nuclear tracers.
Reprinted with permission from Di Rocco RJ, Rumsey WL, Kuczynski BL, et al. Measurement of myocardial blood flow using a coinjection technique for technetium-99m-teboroxine, technetium-96-sestemibi, and Thallium-201. *J Nucl Med.* 1992; 33:1152–1159.

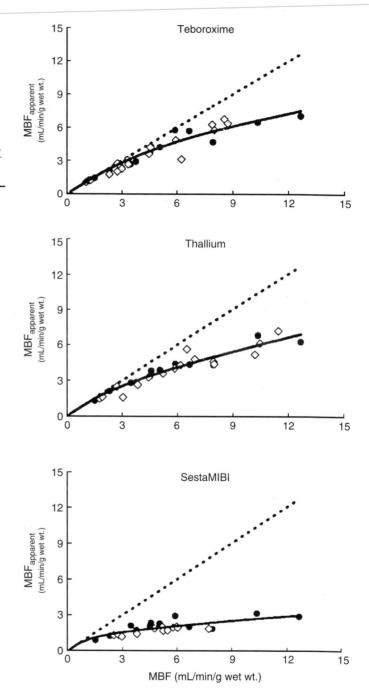

Technetium 99-m Teboroxime (Cardiotec®)
- Boronic acid product.
- Good high flow correlation.
- Drawback: Rapid myocardial clearance (about 10 minutes); therefore, imaging should be done quickly (the lost study phenomenon).
- Redistributes, but because of rapid clearance it cannot be used as viability agent.

- Most of the radioactivity produced by technetium 99-m is gamma ray with an energy level of 140 keV; therefore, the nuclear camera acquisition window should be set around that energy level.

Radiation Safety

1. Biological effects: depend on radiation type, dose, dose rate, and type of tissue. Biological effects are divided into two forms: ***stochastic,*** which does not have a threshold and is cumulative and tends to happen over a long time, for instance, cancer; and ***deterministic,*** which depends on the severity of radiation exposure and has a threshold, for instance, the development of cataract or erythema.
2. ALARA principle: There are certain legal limits of radiation exposure permissible by the Nuclear Regulatory Commission (NRC) (Table 1.1). However, the radiation dose should be kept at ALARA levels (as low as reasonably allowable), even if the ALARA levels are well below the legal levels. In summary, the lower the better.
3. Reducing dose exposure can be achieved by limiting the ***time*** of exposure, increasing ***distance*** from the source (radiation dose decreases inversely with the square of distance, i.e., if you double the distance, the exposure will drop to a quarter of the original exposure), and by ***shielding*** (usually made of lead).
4. The NRC requires that areas with radioactive materials carry labels indicating that there are radioactive materials present and that access to those areas be restricted. Shipments of radioactive materials should be received by a licensee, and detailed records should be kept of the amounts in storage, used, or disposed. Tc-99 and Tl-201 waste should be left to decay until the radiation level is less than twice background.
5. Contamination surveys should be done routinely at the end of each day of use and documented. A spill of less than 1 mCi is called a minor spill, and more than 1 mCi is called a major spill. In case of a spill, access to the area should be restricted immediately. A spill is contained by using liquid absorbent. With any spill more than 1 mCi, the radiation safety officer should be notified immediately, who in turn should notify the NRC.

TABLE 1.1	Current Nuclear Regulatory Commission Maximum Permissible Annual Dose Limit	
		Dose Limit (mSv)
Radiation (occupational) workers		
Total effective dose equivalent limits		50
Dose equivalent limits to tissues and organs		
Lens of eye		150
Skin, hands, and feet		500
Any other organ or tissue		500
General public		
Total effective dose equivalent		1
Embryo-fetus (entire pregnancy)		
Total effective dose equivalent		5

Chandra J. *Nuclear Medicine Physics: The Basics.* 6th ed. Philadelphia, PA: Lippincott Williams and Wilkins; 2006.

FIGURE 1.8 Basic structure of a nuclear camera.

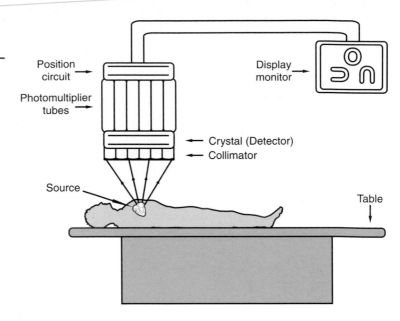

Nuclear SPECT Camera (Scintillation Camera)

The nuclear camera (Figure 1.8) is composed of different parts. Below is a basic description of the different parts and their function:

1. Collimators: Their purpose is to allow X-rays or gamma rays originating from a selected area (the heart, in the case of nuclear cardiology). Collimators are usually made of lead or tungsten. There are many types of collimators, including parallel hole, converging, and diverging. Increasing the field of view reduces the resolution and improves sensitivity.

2. The detector or the crystal: an example is NaI (sodium iodide) crystals, the main function of the crystal is to change the X-rays or gamma rays to light photons (scintillation).

3. Photomultiplier tubes: convert the light photons generated by the NaI crystal to electrons and amplify their energy through applying a high voltage difference. The new generation of cameras made by Digirad® do not have photomultiplier tubes.

4. Position detection circuit: localizes the position of the signal.

5. Display monitor: displays processed myocardial perfusion scans.

REFERENCES

1. Chandra J. *Nuclear Medicine Physics: The Basics.* 6th ed. Philadelphia, PA: Lippincott Williams and Wilkins; 2006.
2. Di Rocco RJ, Rumsey WL, Kuczynski BL, et al. Measurement of myocardial blood flow using a coinjection technique for technetium-99m-teboroxine, technetium-96-sestemibi, and Thallium-201. *J Nucl Med.* 1992; 33: 1152–1159.

Myocardial Perfusion Scans

Indications for Myocardial Perfusion Scans

There has been tremendous growth in the use of myocardial perfusion scans over the years, mainly because of their noninvasive nature, good sensitivity and specificity, and prognostic value. However, in many cases there has been overuse of this technology, leading to unnecessary further testing including invasive procedures, and increasing the cost of health care in general. In 2005, a joint task force of the American College of Cardiology Foundation (ACCF) and the American Society of Nuclear Cardiology (ASNC) published the appropriateness criteria for ordering single photon emission computed tomography (SPECT) myocardial perfusion scans (Tables 2.1–2.12).[1] Following the publication of the appropriateness criteria, the ACCF published a statement of the inappropriate use of SPECT myocardial perfusion imaging (MPI) (Table 2.13). The editors of this book believe that adhering to these criteria leads to the most cost-effective and evidence-based use of this important modality based on the available scientific evidence.

Some of the common indications of stress (exercise or pharmacological) myocardial perfusion scans are:

- Evaluation of chest pain syndrome or acute chest pain
- Evaluation of heart failure and left ventricular systolic function
- Evaluation of ventricular tachycardia
- Evaluation of atrial fibrillation with moderate to high risk
- In patients with valvular heart disease and moderate- and high-risk coronary artery disease (CAD) to help guide decisions of invasive studies
- Evaluation of the physiological importance of coronary stenosis of unclear significance found during coronary angiography
- Worsening symptoms in patients with known CAD
- Patients with non–ST-elevation myocardial infarction (NSTEMI) or troponin elevation when noninvasive management is chosen when making a decision for an invasive study
- Preoperative before noncardiac surgery in moderate- to high-risk patients
- Asymptomatic patients with moderate and high risk for CAD or high-risk occupations
- Patients with high Agatston calcium score greater than or equal to 400
- Patients with stenosis of unclear significance on computed tomography angiography (CTA)
- Patients with borderline stress electrocardiogram (ECG) (without imaging) or nonconclusive stress echocardiogram

TABLE 2.1	Detection of CAD: Symptomatic	
Indication		**Appropriateness Criteria (Median Score)**
Evaluation of Chest Pain Syndrome		
1.	• Low pre-test probability of CAD • ECG interpretable AND able to exercise	**I (2.0)**
2.	• Low pre-test probability of CAD • ECG uninterpretable OR unable to exercise	**U^a (6.5)**
3.	• Intermediate pre-test probability of CAD • ECG interpretable AND able to exercise	**A (7.0)**
4.	• Intermediate pre-test probability of CAD • ECG uninterpretable OR unable to exercise	**A (9.0)**
5.	• High pre-test probability of CAD • ECG interpretable AND able to exercise	**A (8.0)**
6.	• High pre-test probability of CAD • ECG uninterpretable OR unable to exercise	**A (9.0)**
Acute Chest Pain (in Reference to Rest Perfusion Imaging)		
7.	• Intermediate pre-test probability of CAD • ECG—no ST elevation AND initial cardiac enzymes negative	**A (9.0)**
8.	• High pre-test probability of CAD • ECG—ST elevation	**I (1.0)**
New-Onset/Diagnosed Heart Failure With Chest Pain Syndrome		
9.	• Intermediate pre-test probability of CAD	**A (8.0)**

^{a}Median scores of 3.5 and 6.5 are rounded to the middle (Uncertain).
A, (Appropriate); CAD, coronary artery disease; ECG, electrocardiogram; I, (Inappropriate); U, (Uncertain)
Reprinted from Brindis RG, Douglas PS, Hendel RC, et al. ACCF/ASNC appropriateness criteria for single-photon emission computed tomography myocardial perfusion imaging (SPECT MPI): a report of the American College of Cardiology Foundation Quality Strategic Directions Committee Appropriateness Criteria Working Group and the American Society of Nuclear Cardiology endorsed by the American Heart Association. *J Am Coll Cardiol.* 2005; 46:1587–1605, with permission from Elsevier.

TABLE 2.2	Detection of CAD: Asymptomatic (Without Chest Pain Syndrome)	
Indication		**Appropriateness Criteria (Median Score)**
Asymptomatic		
10.	• Low CHD risk (Framingham risk criteria)	**I (1.0)**
11.	• Moderate CHD risk (Framingham)	**U (5.5)**

(*Continued*)

TABLE 2.2	Detection of CAD: Asymptomatic (Without Chest Pain Syndrome) (*Continued*)	
Indication		**Appropriateness Criteria (Median Score)**
New-Onset or Diagnosed Heart Failure or LV Systolic Dysfunction Without Chest Pain Syndrome		
12.	• Moderate CHD risk (Framingham) • No prior CAD evaluation AND no planned cardiac catheterization	A (7.5)
Valvular Heart Disease Without Chest Pain Syndrome		
13.	• Moderate CHD risk (Framingham) • To help guide decision for invasive studies	U (5.5)
New-Onset Atrial Fibrillation		
14.	• Low CHD risk (Framingham) • Part of the evaluation	U[a] (3.5)
15.	• High CHD risk (Framingham) • Part of the evaluation	A (8.0)
Ventricular Tachycardia		
16.	• Moderate to high CHD risk (Framingham)	A (9.0)

[a]Median score of 3.5 and 6.5 are rounded to the middle (Uncertain).
A, (Appropriate); CAD, coronary artery disease; CHD, coronary heart disease; I, (Inappropriate); U, (Uncertain)
Reprinted from Brindis RG, Douglas PS, Hendel RC, et al. ACCF/ASNC appropriateness criteria for single-photon emission computed tomography myocardial perfusion imaging (SPECT MPI): a report of the American College of Cardiology Foundation Quality Strategic Directions Committee Appropriateness Criteria Working Group and the American Society of Nuclear Cardiology endorsed by the American Heart Association. *J Am Coll Cardiol.* 2005; 46:1587–1605, with permission from Elsevier.

TABLE 2.3	Risk Assessment: General and Specific Patient Populations	
Indication		**Appropriateness Criteria (Median Score)**
Asymptomatic		
17.	• Low CHD risk (Framingham)	I (1.0)
18.	• Moderate CHD risk (Framingham)	U (4.0)
19.	• Moderate to high CHD risk (Framingham) • High-risk occupation (e.g., airline pilot)	A (8.0)
20.	• High CHD risk (Framingham)	A (7.5)

A, (Appropriate); CHD, coronary heart disease; I, (Inappropriate); U, (Uncertain)
Reprinted from Brindis RG, Douglas PS, Hendel RC, et al. ACCF/ASNC appropriateness criteria for single-photon emission computed tomography myocardial perfusion imaging (SPECT MPI): a report of the American College of Cardiology Foundation Quality Strategic Directions Committee Appropriateness Criteria Working Group and the American Society of Nuclear Cardiology endorsed by the American Heart Association. *J Am Coll Cardiol.* 2005; 46:1587–1605, with permission from Elsevier.

TABLE 2.4	Risk Assessment With Prior Test Results	
Indication		**Appropriateness Criteria (Median Score)**
Asymptomatic OR Stable Symptoms Normal Prior SPECT MPI Study		
21.	• Normal initial RNI study • High CHD risk (Framingham) • Annual SPECT MPI study	**I (3.0)**
22.	• Normal initial RNI study • High CHD risk (Framingham) • Repeat SPECT MPI study after 2 years or greater	**A (7.0)**
Asymptomatic OR Stable Symptoms Abnormal Catheterization OR Prior SPECT MPI Study		
23.	• Known CAD on catheterization OR prior SPECT MPI study in patients who have not had revascularization procedure • Asymptomatic OR stable symptoms • Less than 1 year to evaluate worsening disease	**I (2.5)**
24.	• Known CAD on catheterization OR prior SPECT MPI study in patients who have not had revascularization procedure • Greater than or equal to 2 years to evaluate worsening disease	**A (7.5)**
Worsening Symptoms Abnormal Catheterization OR Prior SPECT MPI Study		
25.	• Known CAD on catheterization OR prior SPECT MPI study	**A (9.0)**
Asymptomatic CT Coronary Angiography		
26.	• Stenosis of unclear significance	**U[a] (6.5)**
Asymptomatic Prior Coronary Calcium Agatston Score		
27.	• Agatston score greater than or equal to 400	**A (7.5)**
28.	• Agatston score less than 100	**I (1.5)**
UA/NSTEMI, STEMI, or Chest Pain Syndrome Coronary Angiogram		
29.	• Stenosis of unclear significance	**A (9.0)**
Duke Treadmill Score		
30.	• Intermediate Duke treadmill score • Intermediate CHD risk (Framingham)	**A (9.0)**

[a]Median score of 3.5 and 6.5 are rounded to the middle (Uncertain).
A, (Appropriate); CAD, coronary artery disease; CHD, coronary heart disease; I, (Inappropriate); RNI, radionuclide imaging;
SPECT MPI, single photon emission computed tomography myocardial perfusion imaging; U, (Uncertain)
Reprinted from Brindis RG, Douglas PS, Hendel RC, et al. ACCF/ASNC appropriateness criteria for single-photon emission computed tomography myocardial perfusion imaging (SPECT MPI): a report of the American College of Cardiology Foundation Quality Strategic Directions Committee Appropriateness Criteria Working Group and the American Society of Nuclear Cardiology endorsed by the American Heart Association. *J Am Coll Cardiol.* 2005; 46:1587–1605, with permission from Elsevier.

TABLE 2.5   Risk Assessment: Preoperative Evaluation for Noncardiac Surgery

Indication		Appropriateness Criteria (Median Score)
Low–Risk Surgery		
31.	• Preoperative evaluation for noncardiac surgery risk assessment	**I (1.0)**
Intermediate–Risk Surgery		
32.	• Minor to intermediate perioperative risk predictor • Normal exercise tolerance (greater than or equal to 4 METS)	**I (3.0)**
33.	• Intermediate perioperative risk predictor OR • Poor exercise tolerance (less than 4 METS)	**A (8.0)**
High-Risk Surgery		
34.	• Minor perioperative risk predictor • Normal exercise tolerance (greater than or equal to 4 METS)	**U (4.0)**
35.	• Minor Perioperative risk predictor • Poor exercise tolerance (less than 4 METS)	**A (8.0)**
36.	• Asymptomatic up to 1 year post normal catheterization, noninvasive test, or previous revascularization	**I (3.0)**

A, (Appropriate); I, (Inappropriate); METS, metabolic equivalents; U, (Uncertain)
Reprinted from Brindis RG, Douglas PS, Hendel RC, et al. ACCF/ASNC appropriateness criteria for single-photon emission computed tomography myocardial perfusion imaging (SPECT MPI): a report of the American College of Cardiology Foundation Quality Strategic Directions Committee Appropriateness Criteria Working Group and the American Society of Nuclear Cardiology endorsed by the American Heart Association. *J Am Coll Cardiol.* 2005; 46:1587–1605, with permission from Elsevier.

TABLE 2.6   Risk Assessment: Following Acute Coronary Syndrome

Indication		Appropriateness Criteria (Median Score)
STEMI—Hemodynamically Stable		
37.	• Thrombolytic therapy administered • Not planning to undergo catheterization	**A (8.0)**
STEMI—Hemodynamically Unstable, Signs of Cardiogenic Shock, or Mechanical Complications		
38.	• Thrombolytic therapy administered	**I (1.0)**
UA/NSTEMI—No Recurrent Ischemia or No Signs of HF		
39.	• Not planning to undergo early catheterization	**A (8.5)**
ACS —Asymptomatic Post Revascularization (PCI or CABG)		
40.	• Routine evaluation prior to hospital discharge	**I (1.0)**

A, (Appropriate); ACS, acute coronary syndrome; CABG, coronary artery bypass graft; HF, heart failure; I, (Inappropriate); PCI, percutaneous coronary intervention; STEMI, ST-elevation myocardial infarction; U, (Uncertain); UA/NSTEMI, unstable angina/non–ST-elevation myocardial infraction
Reprinted from Brindis RG, Douglas PS, Hendel RC, et al. ACCF/ASNC appropriateness criteria for single-photon emission computed tomography myocardial perfusion imaging (SPECT MPI): a report of the American College of Cardiology Foundation Quality Strategic Directions Committee Appropriateness Criteria Working Group and the American Society of Nuclear Cardiology endorsed by the American Heart Association. *J Am Coll Cardiol.* 2005; 46:1587–1605, with permission from Elsevier.

TABLE 2.7	Risk Assessment-Post-Revascularization (PCI or CABG)	
Indication		**Appropriateness Criteria (Median Score)**
Symptomatic		
41.	• Evaluation of chest pain syndrome	**A (8.0)**
Asymptomatic		
42.	• Asymptomatic prior to previous revascularization • Less than 5 years after CABG	**U (6.0)**
43.	• Symptomatic prior to previous revascularization • Less than 5 years after CABG	**U (4.5)**
44.	• Asymptomatic prior to previous revascularization • Greater than or equal to 5 years after CABG	**A (7.5)**
45.	• Symptomatic prior to previous revascularization • Greater than or equal to 5 years after CABG	**A (7.5)**
46.	• Asymptomatic prior to previous revascularization • Less than 1 year after PCI	**U (6.5)**
47.	• Symptomatic prior to previous revascularization • Less than 1 year after PCI	**1 (3.0)**
48.	• Asymptomatic prior to previous revascularization • Greater than or equal to 2 years after PCI	**U[a] (6.5)**
49.	• Symptomatic prior to previous revascularization • Greater than or equal to 2 years after PCI	**U (5.5)**

[a]Median scores of 3.5 and 6.5 are rounded to the middle (Uncertain).
A, (Appropriate); CABG, coronary artery bypass graft; I, (Inappropriate); PCI, percutaneous coronary intervention; U, (Uncertain)
Reprinted from Brindis RG, Douglas PS, Hendel RC, et al. ACCF/ASNC appropriateness criteria for single-photon emission computed tomography myocardial perfusion imaging (SPECT MPI): a report of the American College of Cardiology Foundation Quality Strategic Directions Committee Appropriateness Criteria Working Group and the American Society of Nuclear Cardiology endorsed by the American Heart Association. *J Am Coll Cardiol.* 2005; 46:1587–1605, with permission from Elsevier.

TABLE 2.8	Assessment of Viability/Ischemia	
Indication		**Appropriateness Criteria (Median Score)**
Ischemic Cardiomyopathy **Assessment of Viability/Ischemia (Includes SPECT Imaging** **for Wall Motion and Ventricular Function)**		
50.	• Known CAD on catheterization • Patient eligible for revascularization	**A (8.5)**

A, (Appropriate); CAD, coronary artery disease; I, (Inappropriate); SPECT, single photon emission computed tomography; U, (Uncertain)
Reprinted from Brindis RG, Douglas PS, Hendel RC, et al. ACCF/ASNC appropriateness criteria for single-photon emission computed tomography myocardial perfusion imaging (SPECT MPI): a report of the American College of Cardiology Foundation Quality Strategic Directions Committee Appropriateness Criteria Working Group and the American Society of Nuclear Cardiology endorsed by the American Heart Association. *J Am Coll Cardiol.* 2005; 46:1587–1605, with permission from Elsevier.

TABLE 2.9	Evaluation of Ventricular Function	
Indication		**Appropriateness Criteria (Median Score)**
Evaluation of Left Ventricular Function		
51.	• Non diagnostic echocardiogram	**A (9.0)**
Use of Potentially Cardiotoxic Therapy (e.g., Doxorubicin)		
52.	• Baseline and serial measurements	**A (9.0)**

A, (Appropriate); I, (Inappropriate); U, (Uncertain)

Reprinted from Brindis RG, Douglas PS, Hendel RC, et al. ACCF/ASNC appropriateness criteria for single-photon emission computed tomography myocardial perfusion imaging (SPECT MPI): a report of the American College of Cardiology Foundation Quality Strategic Directions Committee Appropriateness Criteria Working Group and the American Society of Nuclear Cardiology endorsed by the American Heart Association. *J Am Coll Cardiol.* 2005; 46:1587–1605, with permission from Elsevier.

TABLE 2.10	Inappropriate Indications (Median Rating of 1 to 3)	
Indication		**Appropriateness Criteria (Median Score)**
Detection of CAD: Symptomatic—Evaluation of Chest Pain Syndrome		
1.	• Low pre-test probability of CAD • ECG: interpretable AND able to exercise	**I (2.0)**
Detection of CAD Symptomatic—Acute Chest Pain (in Reference to Rest Perfusion Imaging)		
8.	• High pre-test probability of CAD • ECG: ST elevation	**I (1.0)**
Detection of CAD: Asymptomatic (Without Chest Pain Syndrome)		
10.	• Low CHD risk (Framingham risk criteria)	**I (1.0)**
Risk Assessment: General and Specific Patient Populations—Asymptomatic		
17.	• Low CHD risk (Framingham)	**I (1.0)**
Risk Assessment With Prior Test Results: Asymptomatic OR Stable Symptoms— Normal Prior SPECT MPI Study		
21.	• Normal initial RNI study • High CHD risk (Framingham) • Annual SPECT MPI study	**I (3.0)**
Risk Assessment With Prior Test Results: Asymptomatic OR Stable Symptoms— Abnormal Catheterization OR Prior SPECT MPI Study		
23.	• Known CAD on catheterization OR prior SPECT MPI study in patients who have not had revascularization procedure • Asymptomatic OR stable symptoms • Less than 1 year to evaluate worsening disease	**I (2.5)**
Risk Assessment With Prior Test Results: Asymptomatic—Prior Coronary Calcium Agatston Score		
28.	• Agatston score less than 100	**I (1.5)**

(Continued)

TABLE 2.10	Inappropriate Indications (Median Rating of 1 to 3) (*Continued*)	
Indication		**Appropriateness Criteria (Median Score)**
Risk Assessment: Preoperative Evaluation for Noncardiac Surgery—Low-Risk Surgery		
31.	• Preoperative evaluation for noncardiac surgery risk assessment	**I (1.0)**
Risk Assessment: Preoperative Evaluation for Noncardiac Surgery— Intermediate-Risk Surgery		
32.	• Minor to intermediate perioperative risk predictor • Normal exercise tolerance (greater than or equal to 4 METS)	**I (3.0)**
Risk Assessment: Preoperative Evaluation for Noncardiac Surgery—High Risk Surgery		
36.	• Asymptomatic up to 1 year post normal catheterization, noninvasive test, or previous revascularization	**I (3.0)**
Risk Assessment: Following Acute Coronary Syndrome STEMI—Hemodynamically Unstable, Signs of Cardiogenic Shock, or Mechanical Complications		
38.	• Thrombolytic therapy administered	**I (1.0)**
Risk Assessment: Following Acute Coronary Syndrome— Asymptomatic Post-Revascularization (PCI or CABG)		
40.	• Routine evaluation prior to hospital discharge	**I (1.0)**
Risk Assessment: Post-Revascularization (PCI or CABG)—Asymptomatic		
47.	• Symptomatic prior to previous revascularization • Less than 1 year after PCI	**I (3.0)**

A, (Appropriate); CABG, coronary artery bypass graft; CAD, coronary artery disease; CHD, coronary heart disease; ECG, electrocardiogram; I, (Inappropriate); METS, metabolic equivalents; PCI, percutaneous coronary intervention; RNI, radionuclide imaging; SPECT MPI, single photon emission computed tomography myocardial perfusion imaging; STEMI, ST-elevation myocardial infarction; U, (Uncertain)
Reprinted from Brindis RG, Douglas PS, Hendel RC, et al. ACCF/ASNC appropriateness criteria for single-photon emission computed tomography myocardial perfusion imaging (SPECT MPI): a report of the American College of Cardiology Foundation Quality Strategic Directions Committee Appropriateness Criteria Working Group and the American Society of Nuclear Cardiology endorsed by the American Heart Association. *J Am Coll Cardiol.* 2005; 46:1587–1605, with permission from Elsevier.

TABLE 2.11	Appropriate Indications (Median Rating of 7 to 9)	
Indication		**Appropriateness Criteria (Median Score)**
Detection of CAD): Symptomatic— Evaluation' of Chest Pain Syndrome		
3.	• Intermediate pre-test probability of CAD • ECG interpretable AND able to exercise	**A (7.0)**
4.	• Intermediate pre-test probability of CAD • ECG uninterpretable OR unable to exercise	**A (9.0)**
5.	• High pre-test probability of CAD • ECG interpretable AND able to exercise	**A (8.0)**
6.	• High pre-test probability of CAD • ECG uninterpretable OR unable to exercise	**A (9.0)**

(Continued)

TABLE 2.11	Appropriate Indications (Median Rating of 7 to 9) (*Continued*)	
Indication		**Appropriateness Criteria (Median Score)**
	Detection of CAD: Symptomatic— Acute Chest Pain (in Reference to Rest Perfusion Imaging)	
7.	• Intermediate pre-test probability of CAD • ECG: no ST elevation AND initial cardiac enzymes negative	**A (9.0)**
	Detection of CAD: Symptomatic— New-Onset/Diagnosed Heart Failure With Chest Pain Syndrome	
9.	• Intermediate pre-test probability of CAD	**A (8.0)**
	Detection of CAD: Asymptomatic— New-Onset or Diagnosed Heart Failure of LV Systolic Dysfunction Without Chest Pain Syndrome	
12.	• Moderate CHD risk (Framingham) • No prior CAD evaluation AND no planned cardiac catheterization	**A (7.5)**
	Detection of CAD: Asymptomatic (Without Chest Pain Syndrome)— New-Onset Atrial Fibrillation	
15.	• High CHD Risk (Framingham) • Part of the evaluation	**A (8.0)**
	Detection of CAD: Asymptomatic (Without Chest Pain Syndrome)— Ventricular Tachycardia	
16.	• Moderate to high CHD risk (Framingham)	**A (9.0)**
	Risk Assessment: General and Specific Patient Populations— Asymptomatic	
19.	• Moderate to high CHD risk (Framingham) • High-risk occupation (e.g., airline pilot)	**A (8.0)**
20.	• High CHD risk (Framingham)	**A (7.5)**
	Risk Assessment With Prior Test Results: Asymptomatic OR Stable Symptoms— Normal Prior SPECT MPI Study	
22.	• Normal initial RNI study • High CHD risk (Framingham) • Repeat SPECT MPI study after 2 years or greater	**A (7.0)**
	Risk Assessment With Prior Test Results: Asymptomatic OR Stable Symptoms— Abnormal Catheterization or Prior SPECT MPI Study	
24.	• Known CAD on catheterization OR prior SPECT MPI study in patients who have not had revascularization procedure • Greater than or equal to 2 years to evaluate worsening disease	**A (7.5)**
	Risk Assessment With Prior Test Results: Worsening Symptoms— Abnormal Catheterization OR Prior SPECT MPI Study	
25.	• Known CAD on catheterization OR prior SPECT MPI study	**A (9.0)**

(Continued)

TABLE 2.11	Appropriate Indications (Median Rating of 7 to 9) (*Continued*)	
Indication		**Appropriateness Criteria (Median Score)**
Risk Assessment With Prior Test Results: Asymptomatic— Prior Coronary Calcium Agatston Score		
27.	• Agatston score greater that or equal to 400	**A (7.5)**
Risk Assessment With Prior Test Results: UA/NSTEMI, STEMI, or Chest Pain Syndrome—Coronary Angiogram		
29.	• Stenosis of unclear significance	**A (9.0)**
Risk Assessment With Prior Test Results— Duke Treadmill Score		
30.	• Intermediate Duke treadmill score • Intermediate CHD risk (Framingham)	**A (9.0)**
Risk Assessment: Preoperative Evaluation for Noncardiac Surgery— Intermediate-Risk Surgery		
33.	• Intermediate perioperative risk predictor OR • Poor exercise tolerance (less than 4 METS)	**A (8.0)**
Risk Assessment: Preoperative Evaluation for Noncardiac Surgery— High-Risk Surgery		
35.	• Minor perioperative risk predictor AND • Poor exercise tolerance (less than 4 METS)	**A (8.0)**
Risk Assessment: Following Acute Coronary Syndrome— STEMI-Hemodynamically Stable		
37.	• Thrombolytic therapy administered • Not planning to undergo catheterization	**A(8.0)**
Risk Assessment: Following Acute Coronary Syndrome— UA/NSTEMI—No Recurrent Ischemia OR No Signs of HF		
39.	• Not planning to undergo early catheterization	**A(8.5)**
Risk Assessment: Post-Revascularization (PCI or CABG)— Symptomatic		
41.	• Evaluation of chest pain syndrome	**A(8.0)**
Risk Assessment: Post-Revascularization (PCI or CABG)— Asymptomatic		
44.	• Asymptomatic prior to previous revascularization • Greater than or equal to 5 years after CABG	**A(7.5)**
45.	• Symptomatic prior to previous revascularization • Greater than or equal to 5 years after CABG	**A(7.5)**
Assessment of Viability/Ischemia: Ischemic Cardiomyopathy (Includes SPECT Imaging for Wall Motion and Ventricular Function)		
50.	• Known CAD on catheterization • Patient eligible for revascularization	**A(8.5)**

(Continued)

TABLE 2.11	Appropriate Indications (Median Rating of 7 to 9) (*Continued*)	
Indication		Appropriateness Criteria (Median Score)
Evaluation of Left Ventricular Function		
51.	• Non-diagnostic echocardiogram	**A (9.0)**
Evaluation of Ventricular Function: Use of Potentially Cardiotoxic Therapy (e.g., Doxorubicin)		
52.	• Baseline and serial measurement	**A (9.0)**

A, (Appropriate); CAD, coronary artery disease; CHD, coronary heart disease; ECG, electrocardiogram; I, (Inappropriate); LV, left ventricular; METS, metabolic equivalents; PCI, percutaneous coronary intervention; RNI, radionuclide imaging; STEMI, ST-elevation myocardial infarction; U, (Uncertain); UA/NSTEMI, unstable angina/non–ST-elevation myocardial infarction

Reprinted from Brindis RG, Douglas PS, Hendel RC, et al. ACCF/ASNC appropriateness criteria for single-photon emission computed tomography myocardial perfusion imaging (SPECT MPI): a report of the American College of Cardiology Foundation Quality Strategic Directions Committee Appropriateness Criteria Working Group and the American Society of Nuclear Cardiology endorsed by the American Heart Association. *J Am Coll Cardiol.* 2005; 46:1587–1605, with permission from Elsevier.

TABLE 2.12	Uncertain Indications (Median Rating of 4 to 6) (Possibly Appropriate Indications That Should Be Reimbursed, but Additional Research and/or Patient Information Is Required During Updates of the Criteria in Order to Rate Them Definitively as Being Appropriate)	
Indication		Appropriateness Criteria (Median Score
Detection of CAD: Symptomatic—Evaluation of Chest Pain Syndrome		
2.	• Low pre-test probability of CAD • ECG uninterpretable OR unable to exercise	U[a] (6.5)
Detection of CAD: Asymptomatic (Without Chest Pain Syndrome)		
11.	• Moderate CHD risk (Framingham)	U(5.5)
Detection of CAD: Asymptomatic— Valvular Heart Disease Without Chest Pain Syndrome		
13.	• Moderate CHD risk (Framingham) • To help guide decision for invasive studies	U(5.5)
Detection of CAD: Asymptomatic (Without Chest Pain Syndrome)— New -Onset Atrial Fibrillation		
14.	• Low CHD risk (Framingham) • Part of the evaluation	U[a] (3.5)
Risk Assessment: General and Specific Patient Populations— Asymptomatic		
18.	• Moderate CHD risk (Framingham)	U (4.0)
Risk Assessment With Prior Test Results: Asymptomatic— CT Coronary Angiography		
26.	• Stenosis of unclear significance	U[a] (6.5)

(*Continued*)

TABLE 2.12   Uncertain Indications (Median Rating of 4 to 6) (Possibly Appropriate Indications That Should Be Reimbursed, but Additional Research and/or Patient Information Is Required During Updates of the Criteria in Order to Rate Them Definitively as Being Appropriate) (*Continued*)

Indication		Appropriateness Criteria (Median Score
Risk Assessment: Preoperative Evaluation for Noncardiac Surgery—High-Risk Surgery		
34.	• Minor periopetative risk predictor • Normal exercise tolerance (greater than or equal to 4 METS)	**U (4.0)**
Risk Assessment: Post-Revascularization (PCI or CABG)—Asymptomatic		
42.	• Asymptomatic prior to previous revascularization • Less than 5 years after CABG	**U (6.0)**
43.	• Symptomatic prior to previous revascularization • Less than 5 years after CABG	**U (4.5)**
Risk Assessment: Post-Revascularization (PCI or CABG)—Asymptomatic		
46.	• Asymptomatic prior to previous revascularization • Less than 1 year after PCI	**U[a] (6.5)**
48.	• Asymptomatic prior to previous revascularization • Greater than or equal to 2 years after PCI	**U[a] (6.5)**
49.	• Symptomatic prior to previous revascularization • Greater than or equal to 2 years after PCI	**U (5.5)**

[a]Median scores of 3.5 and 6.5 are rounded to the middle (Uncertain).
A, (Appropriate) CABG, coronary artery bypass graft; CAD, coronary artery disease; CHD, coronary heart disease; ECG, electrocardiogram; I, (Inappropriate); PCI, percutaneous coronary intervention; U, (Uncertain).
Reprinted from Brindis RG, Douglas PS, Hendel RC, et al. ACCF/ASNC appropriateness criteria for single-photon emission computed tomography myocardial perfusion imaging (SPECT MPI): a report of the American College of Cardiology Foundation Quality Strategic Directions Committee Appropriateness Criteria Working Group and the American Society of Nuclear Cardiology endorsed by the American Heart Association. *J Am Coll Cardiol.* 2005; 46:1587–1605, with permission from Elsevier.

TABLE 2.13   Inappropriate Use of SPECT MPI (*Prepare to Justify Your Order for These Indications*)

Today's sophisticated imaging technologies present new possibilities for the cardiovascular patient—and new challenges for the cardiovascular physician, who must decide how best to use them.

The American College of Cardiology Foundation (ACCF) and the American Society of Nuclear Cardiology (ASNC) are leading the way to meet those challenges. The recent publication of the ACCF ASNC Appropriateness Criteria for Single Photon Emission Computed Tomography Myocardial Perfusion Imaging (SPECT MPI) meets a critical need for appropriateness criteria in nuclear cardiovascular imaging. Appropriateness criteria cannot take the place of a physician's best judgment. But they are a critical tool for cardiologists and referring physicians as we strive to avoid overuse of imaging procedures and to practice cost-effective medicine.

(*Continued*)

TABLE 2.13 — Inappropriate Use of SPECT MPI (*Prepare to Justify Your Order for These Indications*) (*Continued*)

A Technical Panel of 12 experts rated the use of SPECT MPI for 52 indications, weighing the risks and benefits of the test in each. Twenty-seven indications were rated appropriate, and 12 were rated possibly appropriate (uncertain). The ACCF and ASNC recommend reimbursement for these 39 indications.

The panel does not recommend reimbursement for the 13 indications rated inappropriate for performing SPECT MPI. When ordering an SPECT MPI for one of the following indications, be aware that payers will likely require additional documentation. Be prepared to justify your order mitigating clinical parameters and patient circumstances.

- **Detection of CAD:** *Evaluation of Chest Pain Syndrome*
  Low pretest probability of CAD, ECG interpretable and able to exercise
- **Detection of CAD:** *Symptomatic Acute Chest Pain (in Reference to Rest Perfusion Imaging)*
  High pretest probability of CAD and ECG: ST elevation
- **Detection of CAD:** *Asymptomatic (without Chest Pain Syndrome)*
  Low CHD Risk based on Framingham Risk Criteria
- **Risk Assessment:** *General and Specific Patient Populations—Asymptomatic*
  Low CHD risk based on Framingham Risk Criteria
- **Risk Assessment with Prior Test Results:** *Asymptomatic or Stable Symptoms—Normal Prior SPECT MPI Study*
  Normal initial RNI study, high CHD risk and annual SPECT MPI study
- **Risk Assessment with Prior Test Results:** *Asymptomatic or Stable Symptoms—Abnormal Catheterization of Prior SPECT MPI Study*
  Known CAD on catheterization or prior SPECT MPI study in patients who have not had revascularization procedure, asymptomatic or stable symptoms, and less than one year to evaluate worsening disease
- **Risk Assessment with Prior Test Results:** *Asymptomatic*
  Prior coronary calcium agatston score less than 100
- **Risk Assessment:** *Preoperative Evaluation for Low-Risk, Noncardiac Surgery* Preoperative evaluation for noncardiac surgery risk assessment
- **Risk Assessment:** *Preoperative Evaluation for Intermediate Risk. Noncardiac Surgery*
  Minor to intermediate perioperative risk predictor and normal exercise tolerance (greater than or equal to 4 METS)
- **Risk Assessment:** *Preoperative Evaluation for High Risk, Noncardiac Surgery* Asymptomatic up to one year post normal catheterization, noninvasive test, or previous revascularization
- **Risk Assessment:** *Following Acute Coronary Syndrome (STEMI—Hemodynamically Unstable, Signs of Cardiogenic Shock, or Mechanical Complications)*
  Thrombolytic therapy administered
- **Risk Assessment: Following Acute Coronary Syndrome**—*Asymptomatic Post Revascularization (PCI or CABG)*
  Routine evaluation prior to hospital discharge
- **Risk Assessment:** *Post-Revascularization, Asymptomatic*
  Symptomatic prior to previous revascularization and less than two years after PCI—pending approval from Technical Panel

BNI, radionuclide imaging; CAD, coronary artery disease; CHD, coronary heart disease; ECG, electrocardiogram; METS, metabolic equivalents
The Appropriateness Criteria for SPECT MPI appear in the Oct 18, 2005, issue of the *Journal of the American College of Cardiology*. 46: 1587–1605. The report is also available at www.acc.org/clinical/pdfs/SPECTMPIACPubFile.pdf.
For additional hard copies. call(800) 253–4636, ext. 8603.
Reprinted from Brindis RG, Douglas PS, Hendel RC, et al. ACCF/ASNC appropriateness criteria for single-photon emission computed tomography myocardial perfusion imaging (SPECT MPI): a report of the American College of Cardiology Foundation Quality Strategic Directions Committee Appropriateness Criteria Working Group and the American Society of Nuclear Cardiology endorsed by the American Heart Association. *J Am Coll Cardiol.* 2005; 46:1587–1605, with permission from Elsevier.

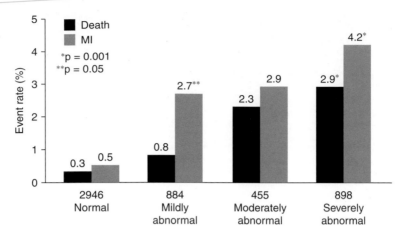

FIGURE 2.1 Cardiac death and myocardial infarction rates related to SPECT perfusion scan results. MI, myocardial infarction; SPECT, single photon emission computed tomography.
Reprinted with permission from Hachamovitch R, Hayes SW, Friedman JD, Cohen I, Berman DS. Comparison of the short-term survival benefit associated with revascularization compared with medical therapy in patients with no prior coronary artery disease undergoing stress myocardial perfusion single photon emission computed tomography. *Circulation* 2003; 107:2900–2907.

The Prognostic Value of Myocardial Perfusion Imaging

One of the big advantages of myocardial perfusion scans is their prognostic value, which has been established in multiple studies (Figure 2.1).[2–6] In addition, the degree of the abnormality of the myocardial perfusion scan can help in decision making whether the patient should undergo revascularization versus medical management. It has been shown that patients with normal scans or with defects less than 10% of the myocardium who underwent revascularization had higher mortality than those who had medical management (Figure 2.2).[7]

FIGURE 2.2 Mortality related to ischemic defect size and medical therapy versus revascularization. Reprinted with permission from Hachamovitch R, Berman DS, Kiat H, et al. Incremental prognostic value of Adenosine stress myocardial perfusion single-photon emission computed tomography and impact on subsequent management in patients with or suspected of having myocardial ischemia. *Am J Cardiol.* 1997; 80:426–433.

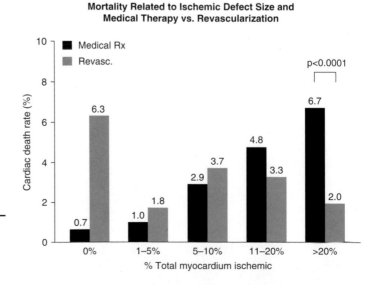

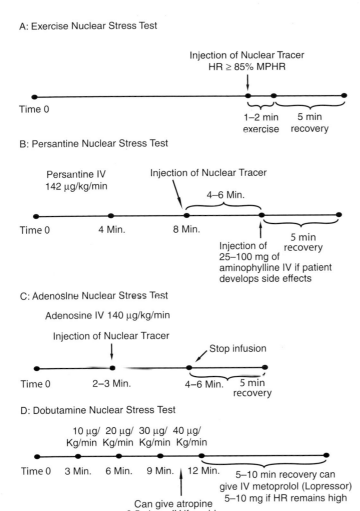

FIGURE 2.3 Different protocols of exercise and pharmacological stress testing. HR, heart rate; IV, intravenous; MPHR, maximum predicted heart rate.

Types of Stress Tests and Different Protocols

There are many protocols for performing myocardial perfusion imaging, each having its indications, advantages, and disadvantages (Figure 2.3).

Exercise Stress Test Myocardial Perfusion Scan

This should be the standard form of stress test if the patient is able to exercise and in the absence of left bundle branch block. It has many advantages over the other modalities of stress tests. The most commonly used stress test protocol is the standard Bruce protocol, which has many advantages:

- It has a prognostic value through the calculation of the Duke score. Duke score = (exercise time in minutes) − (5 × ST change) − (4 × angina index). 0 = no angina, 1 = angina induced during stress test, 2 = treadmill stopped due to angina. A Duke score greater than or equal to 5 has the best survival (4-year survival of 99%, 7-year survival of 95%). A score of −10 to +4 has a 4-year survival rate of 95% and a 7-year survival rate of 91%. A score of less than or equal to −11 carries the worst prognosis (4-year survival of 79% and 7-year survival of 78%) .
- It evaluates arrythmias and chrontotropic incompetence.

TABLE 2-14	Contraindications to Exercise Testing

Absolute
- Acute Myocardial infarction (within 2 d)
- High-risk unstable angina
- Uncontrolled cardiac arrhythmias causing symptoms of hemodynamic compromise
- Symptomatic severe aortic stenosis
- Uncontrolled symptomatic heart failure
- Acute pulmonary embolus or pulmonary infarction
- Acute myocarditis or pericarditis
- Acute aortic dissection

Relative
- Left main coronary stenosis
- Moderate stenotic valvular heart disease
- Electrolyte abnormalities
- Severe arterial hypertension
- Tachyarrhythmias or bradyarrhythmias
- Hypertrophic cardiomyopathy and other forms of outflow trace obstruction
- Mental or physical impairment leading to inability to exercise adequately
- High-degree atrioventricular block

ACA/AHA Guidelines for the management of patients with unstable angina/non-STsegment elevation myocardial infarction. Reprinted from Brindis RG, Douglas PS, Hendel RC, et al. ACCF/ASNC appropriateness criteria for single-photon emission computed tomography myocardial perfusion imaging (SPECT MPI): a report of the American College of Cardiology Foundation Quality Strategic Directions Committee Appropriateness Criteria Working Group and the American Society of Nuclear Cardiology endorsed by the American Heart Association. *J Am Coll Cardiol.* 2005; 46:1587–1605, with permission from Elsevier.

During the exercise stress test the patient should be injected with the stress dose of the nuclear tracer at peak exercise, and then the patient should be allowed to exercise for about one minute.

It should be kept in mind that the exercise stress test has absolute and relative contraindications (Table 2.14),[8] and therefore careful history taking and a focused physical exam should be performed before beginning the stress test.

Dipyridamole (Persantine) Stress Test

Dipyridamole is a vasodilator. It acts by inhibiting cellular uptake of Adenosine, leading to the accumulation of Adenosine, which leads to vasodilation. Dipyridamole is usually infused for a total duration of 4 minutes at a rate of 142 μg/kg per minute. It is usually indicated as an alternative to the exercise stress test in patients who cannot exercise. The stress dose of the nuclear tracer should be injected at 4 minutes post dipyridamole infusion. The patient may develop side effects including flushing, nausea, headache, atrioventricular (AV) block, or bronchospasm. These side effects can be reversed by injecting aminophylline (25–100 mg) intravenously.

Persantine is contraindicated in patients with bronchospastic airway disease or high grade AV block.

Adenosine Stress Test

Adenosine is an active short-acting metabolite that works as a strong vasodilator. It has the same indications as the Persantine stress test; however, it is much shorter acting (half-life of Adenosine is about 6–10 seconds compared to that of intravenous Persantine, which is about 25 minutes). There are many protocols for Adenosine infusion where Adenosine is infused at a rate of 140 μg/kg per minute for a total duration of 4–6 minutes. The stress dose of nuclear tracer is injected at the third minute of the Adenosine infusion. Adenosine has similar side effects compared to Persantine, with more severe AV block episodes. However, the side effects of Adenosine are short lived because of its very short half-life.

Both Adenosine and dipyridamole are vasodilators and will induce more vasodilation in normal or less stenotic arteries compared to coronaries with severe stenosis, leading to relative differential vasodilation (more in normal vessels and less in stenotic vessels) and hence to differential tracer uptake, which helps determine areas of less myocardial blood flow.

It should be kept in mind that patients undergoing Persantine or Adenosine stress tests should abstain from caffeine-containing products as well as aminophylline or theophylline for 24 hours, since these products block Adenosine receptors.

Lexiscon© (regadenoson) Stress Test

Regadenoson is an A_{2A} receptors agonist with 10-fold lower affinity to A_1 receptors and weak if any affinity to A_{2B} & A_3 Adenosine receptors. It has been very recently introduced to the U.S. market. It is contraindicated in second or third degree AV Block or sinus node dysfunction.

The protocol of adminstration as directed by the manufacturer involves the administration of 0.4 mg/5mL single viral, followed immediately by 5 ml saline flush then adminstering the radionuclide imaging agent 10–20 seconds after the saline flush.

Multicenter study showed that regodenoson provides diagnostic information compared to a standard Adenosine infusion.[9] Due to the recent introduction of this pharmacological agent, the clinical experience associated with its use remains limited.

Dobutamine Stress Test

This is usually used in patients who cannot exercise and cannot tolerate Persantine or Adenosine, mainly due to severe obstructive airway disease. Dobutamine is infused at a rate of 10 μg/kg per minute with a 10 μg/kg per minute increase every 3 minutes to a maximum dose of 40 μg/kg per minute. Atropine (up to 1 mg intravenously in divided dose) may be added to achieve target heart rate. The stress dose of nuclear tracer is usually given at peak heart rate. Low dose, short-acting β blockers (such as metoprolol, 5 mg) may be given during recovery. Dobutamine has the same contraindications as exercise stress testing with extra precautions in cases of ventricular arrhythmias.

Perfusion Scan Layout and Definitions

The perfusion scan layout varies depending on the software used. However, it has been the standard to display the scans in three views:

1. Cross sectional: The slices are usually displayed from the apex (left) to the base (right).
2. Vertical long axis: The slices are displayed from the septal area (left) to the lateral (right).
3. Horizontal long axis: The slices are usually displayed from the inferior portion (left) to the superior portion (right).

It is the convention to put the stress images on the top row with the corresponding rest images in the lower row to facilitate the comparison.

Each of the sections described above help in evaluating certain areas of the myocardium, and combing the information from all sections gives a comprehensive idea about the perfusion of the whole myocardium (Figure 2.4).

It should be noted that the SPECT segments correspond to certain coronary distributions in general; however, many exceptions should be noted, keeping in mind the wide variability in coronary anatomy among humans. The dominant left circumflex artery usually takes the distribution of the right coronary artery in addition to the usual areas supplied by the left

FIGURE 2.4 Layouts and angiographic correlations of myocardial perfusion scans. LAD, left anterior descending artery; LC$_X$, left circumflex artery; RCA, right coronary artery.

A. CROSS SECTIONS

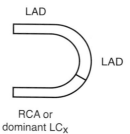

Apex   Mid Anterior   Basal Anterior

B. VERTICAL LONG AXIS

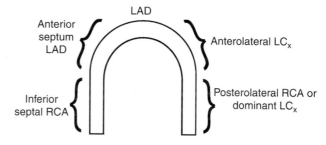

C. HORIZONTAL LONG AXIS

circumflex. A large left anterior descending artery may wrap around the apex to variable degrees, and hence could supply variable parts of the inferior apex and the inferior wall. On the other hand, a very large right coronary artery could supply part of the apex and parts of the anterior apical areas usually supplied by the left anterior descending artery.

With the growing number of patients with coronary artery bypass surgery, it should always be kept in mind that two vessels could supply certain areas on a perfusion scan. For example, in cases of left internal mammary artery (LIMA) graft to native mid left anterior descending artery (LAD), the distal anterior and apical areas are supplied by the LIMA graft while the anterior basal and mid anterior are supplied by the native LAD, and it is not unusual to see infarction or ischemia in those area caused by native vessel disease.

The Normal Scan, Infarction, and Ischemia

The normal scan is characterized by homogenous tracer uptake in both the stress and rest images without perfusion defects or significant artifacts, and without transient ischemic dilation. The left ventricle should be normal in size and the gated images should reveal normal systolic function with ejection fraction equal to or greater than 50% with normal wall motion (Figure 2.5). A normal nuclear scan should be obtained at an adequate workload greater than or equal to 85% of maximum predicted heart rate (MPHR) or with a pharmacological stress protocol.

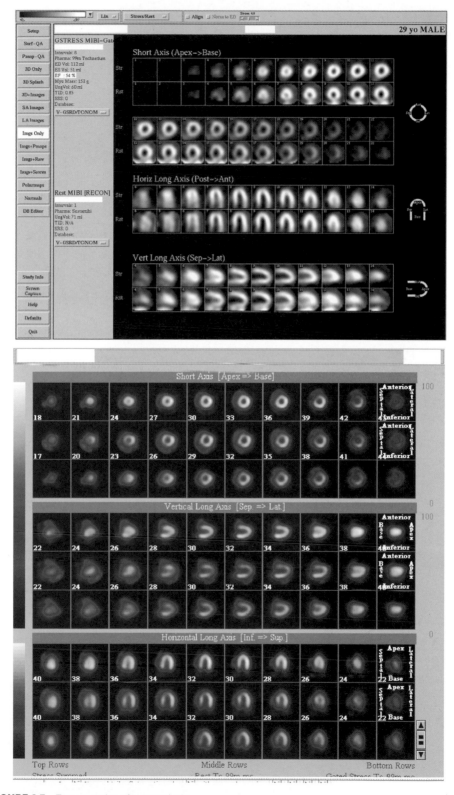

FIGURE 2.5 Two examples of a normal scan.

Infarction

Infarction is a fixed defect in both the stress and rest images that does not fill in the gated images. Infarction could be complete when there is no tracer activity at all, or partial when there is some tracer activity. An infarcted area is usually associated with wall motion abnormality in that area.

Ischemia

Ischemia is characterized by reduced tracer activity during stress in certain area(s), reflecting reduced blood flow that has normal or improved tracer activity in the rest images.

Angiographic Correlation

As discussed above, there are certain myocardial perfusion scan patterns that correlate with significant stenosis in each of the coronary arteries. Below are examples with explanations to demonstrate these angiographic correlations.

Left Anterior Descending Artery Disease

This is characterized by abnormal tracer activity in the apex, anterior wall, and the septal area if the stenosis is in the proximal portion of the LAD before the origin of the septal branch (Figure 2.6).

The scans in Figure 2.6 are of a 65-year-old male who presented with typical chest pain. The patient underwent an exercise myocardial perfusion scan. He exercised 10 minutes and 20 seconds and then stopped because of chest pain and ST depression. Maximum heart rate (HR) was 131 (84% predicted). Maximum blood pressure (BP) was 150/84. The scans demonstrate a reduction of tracer activity in the anterior, apical, and septal areas that improves during rest, indicating ischemia in the LAD territory.

Based on the above findings, the patient was referred to cardiac catheterization and was found to have severe stenosis of the proximal portion of the LAD and had a successful percutaneous intervention.

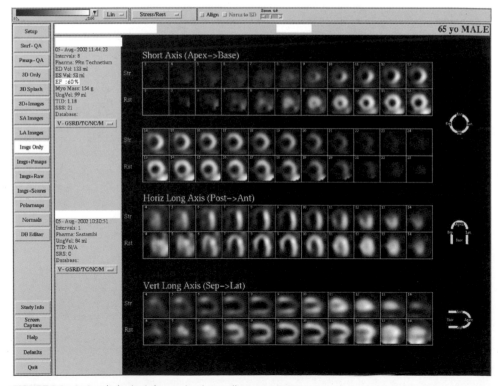

FIGURE 2.6 Ischemia in the left anterior descending artery area.

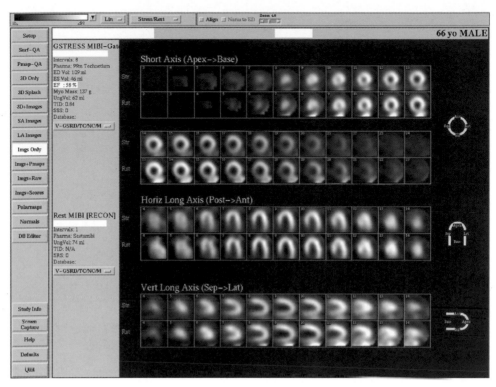

FIGURE 2.7   Same patient in Figure 2.6 after percutaneous intervention to the left anterior descending artery.

The patient returned 1 month later for a follow-up stress test. He exercised for 12 minutes and achieved 91% MPHR without chest pain. The stress ECG was negative for ischemia, and the new myocardial perfusion was within normal limits (Figure 2.7).

Left Circumflex Disease

Left circumflex disease usually manifests as perfusion abnormalities in the lateral wall (Figure 2.8). However, the abnormality could also involve the inferior wall in cases of left dominant systems where the circumflex supplies the inferior wall.

Right Coronary Artery Disease

Right coronary artery disease usually manifests as inferior defects that could involve the inferior apical area and the inferoseptal areas (Figure 2.9).

Diagonal Branch Disease

Diagonal branch disease usually presents as a perfusion abnormality involving the distal anterior and apical lateral areas sparing the apex itself, which is usually supplied by the left anterior descending artery (Figure 2.10).

Balanced Ischemia

Balanced ischemia is the Achilles' heal of SPECT myocardial perfusion scans, usually because of multi-vessel disease where there is a reduction of tracer activity in all vascular territories, making it difficult to appreciate ischemia. Findings that could raise suspicion of balanced ischemia are chest pain during stress test, drop in blood pressure during stress test, and abnormal electrocardiogram. On the perfusion scans, transient ischemic dilation (TID) and reduced left ventricular systolic function on the gated images should raise suspicion about balanced ischemia in light of

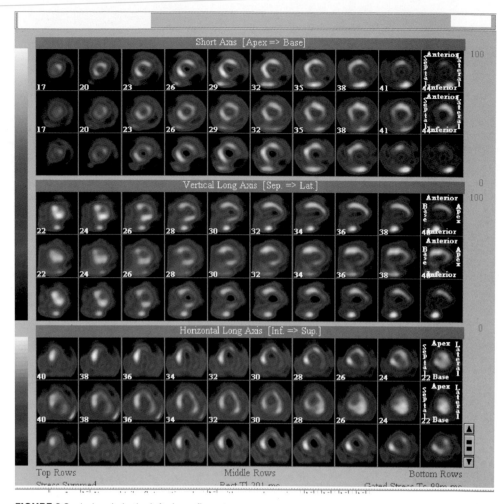

FIGURE 2.8   Ischemia in the left circumflex artery area.

the absence of regional perfusion abnormalities (Figure 2.11). Finally, measuring myocardial perfusion scans using positron emission tomography can accurately detect significant multi-vessel disease with high sensitivity, as discussed in another chapter of this book.

Ischemic Cardiomyopathy

Ischemic cardiomyopathy (CMP) usually presents as an enlarged left ventricle with a large infarcted and ischemic area that correlates to one or more vascular territories (Figure 2.12).

Left Ventricle Aneurysm

This is usually associated with ischemic cardiomyopathy presentation and is characterized by the diversion of the anterior and inferior walls and septal and lateral walls.

Non-ischemic Cardiomyopathy

Non-ischemic cardiomyopathy usually presents as an enlarged ventricle with heterogeneous tracer uptake involving more than one vascular territory, without a clear area of large infarction. In many cases it could be confused with inferior infarction because the enlarged left ventricle tends to extend inferiorly and therefore has more diaphragmatic attenuation. Gated

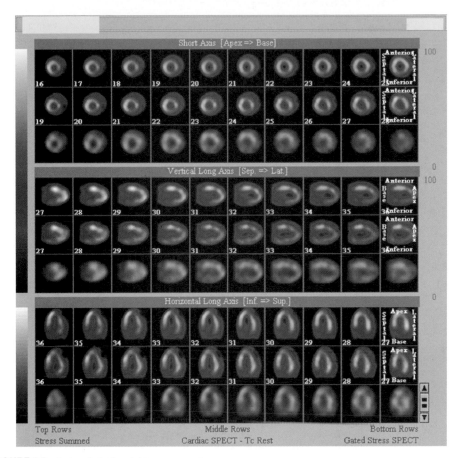

FIGURE 2.9 Ischemia in the right coronary artery area.

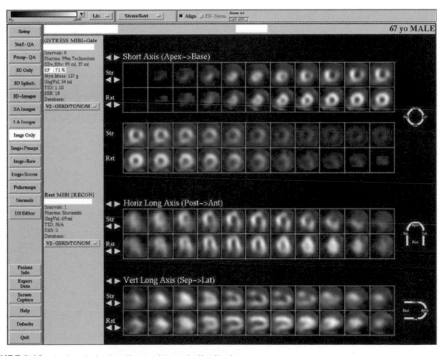

FIGURE 2.10 Ischemia in the diagonal branch distribution.

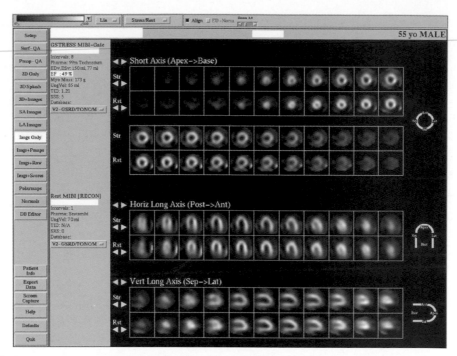

FIGURE 2.11 Balanced ischemia with transient ischemic dilation.

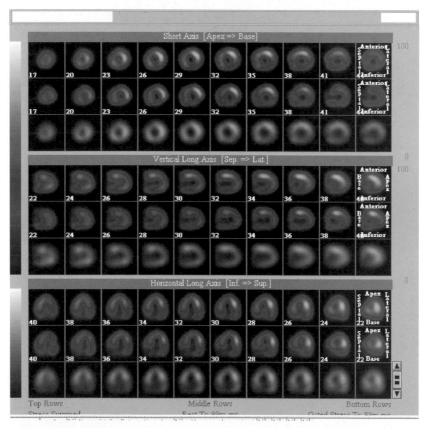

FIGURE 2.12 Ischemic cardiomyopathy with dilated left ventricle and infarction in the left anterior descending artery and right coronary artery territories.

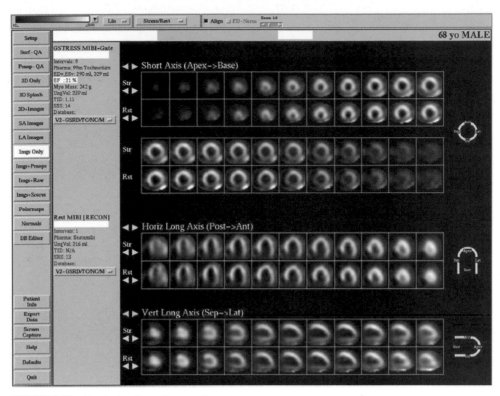

FIGURE 2.13   Non-ischemic cardiomyopathy.

studies usually help by showing global hypokinesis. In all cases, the SPECT images have limited accuracy in distinguishing ischemic from non-ischemic cardiomyopathy, and in most cases patients will require cardiac catheterization or CT angiography if the clinical presentation is highly suggestive of non-ischemic CMP (Figure 2.13).

Congenital Anomalies of the Coronary Arteries

Nuclear cardiology studies are not the best way to diagnose congenital anomalies of coronary arteries where other available techniques (such as cardiac magnetic resonance angiography [MRA], cardiac computed tomography angiography [CTA], or cardiac catheterization) can give accurate anatomic information about these anomalies. However, SPECT images can give an idea about the physiologic significance of such anomalies and help in choosing management strategies. Figure 2.14 is of 26-year-old woman who was diagnosed with anomalous left coronary artery from the pulmonary artery (ALCAPA). The nuclear stress test showed anterior ischemia and the patient underwent single-vessel coronary artery bypass surgery.

Gating and Ejection Fraction Calculation

Gating represents a major advance in nuclear cardiology, making it possible to calculate ejection fraction (EF), which carries major prognostic significance and is the strongest predictor of outcomes.[10] It also helps to differentiate infarctions from soft-tissue attenuation. Attenuated areas tend to thicken normally in the gated images, while infarcted areas remain as fixed defects in the gated images associated with wall motion abnormalities. The following points should be kept in mind in evaluating ejection fraction obtained from gated SPECT images:

- SPECT ejection fraction is not accurate in cases of gross rhythm irregularities such atrial fibrillation or frequent ectopy.

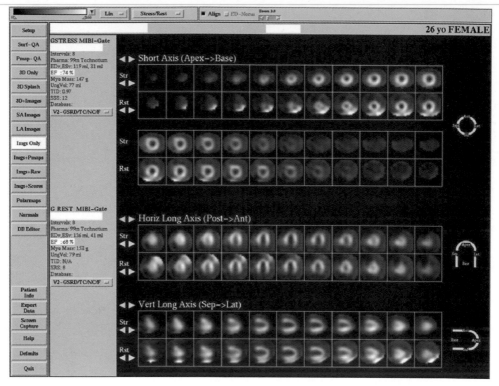

FIGURE 2.14 Myocardial perfusion scan in a case of anomalous left coronary artery from the pulmonary artery syndrome.

- Gating and ejection fraction are usually calculated from post-stress images, and therefore a low ejection fraction in the absence of perfusion defects should raise suspicion of balanced ischemia.
- Most of the SPECT software systems tend to overestimate ejection fraction in small hearts and underestimate it in large hearts.
- In general, SPECT-derived EF correlates well with that obtained from other modalities such as echocardiogram, magnetic resonance imaging (MRI), and left ventriculography.

Artifacts

Artifacts represent the major limitation for SPECT that limits the sensitivity and specificity of this technique. There are many sources of artifacts. Each artifact has a certain pattern, and there are certain steps to limit the impact of these artifacts on the quality of the study; but in some cases it is not possible to eliminate them completely. The best strategy to limit artifacts is by preventing them during the acquisition of the nuclear scans. It is also very important to review the raw images (rotatograms) as part of the study because most of the artifacts will be noted.

Types of SPECT artifacts include:

- Breast attenuation: This is the most common artifact in women and it presents as antero-apical septal thinning in both stress and rest images that usually thickens normally in the gated images. Breast shadows can be noted in raw images (rotatograms).
- Diaphragmatic attenuation: This usually presents as inferior thinning that thickens normally in the gated images. Diaphragm shadow may be noted on the raw images.

- Motion artifact: This may be easily noted on the raw images, and the motion artifact may be horizontal or vertical. Some image processing software systems offer auto-correction of the motion artifacts, but in many cases motion artifacts may affect the interpretation of the study. The best solution to motion artifacts is to prevent them by giving clear instructions to the patient, and in some cases reacquisition of the images is needed.
- Intestinal uptake: This usually affects the inferior wall and could lead to the false diagnosis of inferior ischemia. It occurs more with vasodilator agents such as Persantine or Adenosine because of splanchnic vasodilation. Intestinal activity may overlap with the inferior wall and it may become difficult to separate them from each other. Potential solutions include:

  - Waiting 45–60 minutes after the stress test before image acquisition
  - Reprocessing the images with careful exclusion of the intestines
  - Offering a drink or a snack post stress test
  - Asking the patient to perform minor exercise (such as walking on the treadmill at zero angle) while infusing the vasodilator

Attenuation Correction

Soft-tissue attenuation remains one of the biggest limitations to SPECT imaging, and overcoming such limitations will greatly enhance the accuracy of this imaging modality. Multiple attempts to establish attenuation correction protocols and algorithms have been tried in different studies with variable degrees of success.[11–14] However, there are many limitations to this technology, such as having more false results in the apical area and truncation artifacts. In addition, attenuation correction requires additional hardware and software, and extra time for image processing. All these factors have limited the routine use of attenuation correction in light of the absence of solid evidence of its advantage. The editors of this book recommend a wait and see position regarding this technology until the development of software and hardware capable of complete attenuation correction is verified by large studies.

Lung Uptake

Increased lung uptake and hence lung–heart ratio (LHR), especially in Thallium stress tests, is known to be a sign of multi-vessel heart disease and carries poor prognosis. It is usually measured by placing a region of interest on the lung, then on the myocardium, and comparing the two. The LHR is of less value in Technetium-based studies, the scans are performed 30–60 minutes post injection which gives time to the tracer to clear from the lungs. However, some studies have shown that sestamibi lung–heart ratio can predict outcomes similar to Thallium lung uptake.[15]

Polar Maps

A polar map is a plot of tracer activity in all short axis slices, with the apex in the center and basal slices in the outer rings. Stress images are on top and rest images are on the bottom. The maps are constructed in the classic "bull's eye" fashion. An additional blackout polar map is also used, indicating the extent of perfusion defect by blackening the area of myocardium that is less than 2.5 SD below sex-specific normal database comparison.[16] Polar maps have many limitations, and their results should not be the sole source of scan interpretation; however, they should be routinely reviewed to draw attention to any perfusion abnormalities that were overlooked in the visual interpretation of scans.

Neural Networks in Nuclear Cardiology

Neural networks are computer-based programs that are built in a way to simulate cerebral processing. They are trained by a certain set of data and are used to make decisions (diagnoses) using input data. Artificial neural networks have been increasingly used in different fields of radiology.[17,18] Recently it was shown that computer-based neural networks that integrate clinical data and exercise stress test data, as well as myocardial perfusion scan data can perform as well as expert readers in diagnosing coronary artery disease.[19]

Sensitivity and Specificity of SPECT

Multiple studies have been performed to address the sensitivity and specificity of this commonly used technology. Exercise myocardial perfusion scans have an average sensitivity and specificity of 87% and 73%, respectively, (Table 2.15), with 89% and 75%, respectively, for vasodilator myocardial perfusion scans (Table 2.16).[16] However, it should be kept in mind that these studies are limited by many factors, including referral bias. The other important factor is that myocardial perfusion imaging (a physiological test) is compared to cardiac catheterization (an anatomical test), which evaluates the lumen of coronary arteries and hence has the limitation of missing diffuse disease. In some instances, endothelial dysfunction, especially in diabetics, can cause perfusion abnormality that can't be demonstrated in cardiac catheterization. Further controversy arises when knowing that borderline lesions found during cardiac catheterization are further evaluated using specialized catheter-based techniques such as intravascular ultrasound (IVUS) and fractional flow reserve (FFR), both of which have been validated using myocardial perfusion scans as the gold standard.[20]

Stress Test and Myocardial Perfusion Imaging Report

There is more than one way of reporting the MPI findings. The American Society of Nuclear Cardiology (ASNC) published a document that can be found on the ASNC Web site (see Appendix 1) and may be very helpful in establishing a successful reporting system. The ASNC document is in favor of a standardized reporting system and strongly encourages clarity of reports.

The editors realize that there is more than one reporting format but strongly encourage consideration of the following:

1. It is preferable to have one combined report for both the stress test and myocardial perfusion scan since the findings of these tests are complimentary to each other. In addition, it is more efficient and time saving to combine both reports in one, and it makes it easier for the referring physician to get a clear idea about the results of both these tests.

2. The first portion should include the patient's identifying information, including name, age, gender, and date of birth. It is also very important to include the patient's weight. Both the gender and weight are important in evaluating sources of artifacts.

3. History and indication: This should include a brief history of the patient's risk factors and the indications for the test.

4. Stress test: This section contains a description of the stress test, whether exercise or pharmaceutical, with a description of the protocol, duration, symptoms, reason for stopping the test, heart rate at baseline, and, with exercise stress tests, baseline ECG, stress ECG, and arrhythmia. In pharmacological stress tests, the infusion dose and its duration should be mentioned. The timing of the stress dose of nuclear tracer in

			Prior	Sensitivity		Specificity	
Year	Author	Radiopharmaceutical	MI (%)	Pts. with CAD	%	Pts. w/out CAD	%
2001	Elhendy	Sestamibi Tetrofosmin	0	183/240	76	67/92	73
1999	Azzarelli	Tetrofosmin	66	199/209	95	20/26	77
1998	San Roman	Sestamibi	0	54/62	87	21/30	70
1998	Budoff	Sestamibi	0	12/16	75	12/17	71
1998	Santana-Boado	Sestamibi	0	91/100	91	57/63	90
1998	Acampa	Sestamibi	47	23/25	92	5/7	71
1998	Acampa	Tetrofosmin	47	24/25	96	6/7	86
1998	Ho	Tl-201	22	19/24	79	15/20	75
1997	Iskandrian	Tl-201	21	717/820	87	120/173	69
1997	Candell-Riera	Sestamibi	0	53/57	93	32/34	94
1997	Yao	Sestamibi	55	34/36	94	14/15	93
1997	Heiba	Sestamibi	31	28/30	93	2/4	50
1997	Ilo	Tl-201	33	29/38	76	10/13	77
1997	Taillefer	Sestamibi	17	23/32	72	13/16	81
1997	Van Eck-Smit	Tetrofosmin	NR	46/53	87	6/7	86
1996	Hambye	Sestamibi	0	75/91	82	28/37	75
1995	Palmas	Sestamibi	30	60/66	91	3/4	75
1995	Rubello	Sestamibi	57	100/107	93	8/13	61
1994	Sylven	Sestamibi	37	41/57	72	5/10	50
1994	Van Train	Sestamibi	19	91/102	89	8/22	36
1993	Berman	Sestamibi/Tl-201	0	50/52	96	9/11	82
1993	Forster	Sestamibi	0	10/12	83	8/9	89
1993	Chae	Tl-201	42	116/163	71	52/80	65
1993	Mmoves	Sestamibi/Tl-201	42	27/30	90	22/24	92
1993	Van Train	Sestamibi	16	30/31	97	6/9	67
1992	Quinones	Tl-201	NR	65/86	76	21/26	81
1991	Coyne	Tl-201	NR	38/47	81	39/53	74
1991	Pozzoli	Sestamibi	19	41/49	84	23/26	88
1990	Kiat	Sestamibi	45	45/48	94	4/5	80
1990	Mahmarian	Tl-201	43	192/221	87	65/75	87
1990	Nguyen	Tl-201	NR	19/25	75	5/5	100
1990	Van Train	Tl-201	35	291/307	95	30/64	47
1989	Iskandrian	Tl-201	45	145/164	88	36/58	62
	Total			2971/3425		772/1055	
	Average				87		73

TABLE 2.15 Sensitivity and Specificity of Exercise Myocardial Perfusion Single Photon Emission Computed Tomography for Detecting Coronary Artery Disease (Greater Than or Equal to 50% Stenosis)—Generally Without Correction for Referral Bias

MI, myocardial infarction; NR, not reported; Sestamibi, Tc-99m-sestamibi; Tetrofosmin Tc-99m-tetrofosmin; Tl-201, tinallium-201.

Based on English language manuscripts providing data with greater than or equal to 50% stenosis criterion.

Reprinted from Brindis RG, Douglas PS, Hendel RC, et al. ACCF/ASNC appropriateness criteria for single-photon emission computed tomography myocardial perfusion imaging (SPECT MPI): a report of the American College of Cardiology Foundation Quality Strategic Directions Committee Appropriateness Criteria Working Group and the American Society of Nuclear Cardiology endorsed by the American Heart Association. *J Am Coll Cardiol.* 2005; 46:1587–1605, with permission from Elsevier.

TABLE 2.16 Sensitivity and Specificity of Vasodilator Stress Single-Photon Emission Computed Tomography for Detecting Coronary Aretery Disease (Greater Than or Equal to 50% Stenosis)—Without Correction for Referral Bias

Year	Author	Vasodilator	Radiopharmaceutical	Prior MI (%)	Sensitivity Pts with CAD	%	Specificity Pts w/out CAD	%
2000	Smart	Dipyridamole	Sestamibi	NR	95/119	80	47/64	73
1998	Takeishi	Adenosine	Tetrofosmin	17	39/44	89	17/21	81
1997	Watanabe	Adenosine	Tl-201	19	40/46	87	21/24	88
1997	Watanabe	Dipyridamole	Tl-201	23	34/41	83	21/29	72
1997	Taillefer	Dipyridamole	Sestamibi	11	23/32	72	5/5	100
1997	He	Dipyridamole	Tetrofosmin	52	41/48	85	6/11	55
1997	Cuocolo	Adenosine	Tetrofosmin	23	22/25	88	1/1	100
1997	Amanullah	Adenosine	Sestamibi/Tl-201	0	159/171	93	37/51	73
1997	Miller	Dipyridamole	Sestamibi	34	186/204	91	11/40	28
1997	Iskandrian	Adenosine	Tl-201	28	452/501	90	41/49	84
1995	Aksut	Adenosine	Tl-201	24	358/398	90	38/45	84
1995	Miyagawa	Adenosine	Tl-201	15	67/76	88	35/44	80
1993	Marwick	Adenosine	Sestamibi	0	51/59	86	27/38	71
1991	Coyne	Adenosine	Tl-201	NR	39/47	83	40/53	75
1991	Nishimura	Adenosine	Tl-201	13	61/70	87	28/31	90
1990	Verani	Adenosine	Tl-201	NR	24/29	83	15/16	94
1990	Nguyen	Adenosine	Tl-201	37	49/53	92	7/7	100
	Total				1740/1963		397/529	
	Average					89		75

Based on English language manuscripts providing data with ≤ 50% stenosis criterion.

MI, myocardial infarction; NR, not reported; Sestamibi; Tc-99m-sestamibi; Tetrofosmin, Tc-99m-tetrofosmin; Tl-201, Thallium-201.

Reprinted from Brindis RG, Douglas PS, Hendel RC, et al. ACCF/ASNC appropriateness criteria for single-photon emission computed tomography myocardial perfusion imaging (SPECT MPI); a report of the American College of Cardiology Foundation Quality Strategic Directions Committee Appropriateness Criteria Working Group and the American Society of Nuclear Cardiology endorsed by the American Heart Association. *J Am Coll Cardiol.* 2005; 46:1587–1605, with permission from Elsevier.

relation to the stress test should be mentioned, e.g., at peak exercise or 2 minutes after starting the Adenosine infusion.

5. Myocardial perfusion scan findings: Study quality and limitations (if any) should be stated first. A detailed description of the tracer activity should be mentioned, including segments with the abnormalities, the severity of abnormality, and reversibility. Gated images should be thoroughly described, including the size of the left ventricle, ejection fraction, and wall motion description. Any abnormality of the right ventricle should also be mentioned, such as wall hypertrophy or enlargement.

6. Impression or conclusion: This is the most important part of the report and should include clear sentences that will help the referring physician to make management decisions. This section should include the following: (a) results of the stress test; (b) limitations (if any) of the myocardial perfusion scans; (c) results of the myocardial perfusion scans (normal, abnormal, or borderline); (d) type, size, and severity of abnormalities; (g) gated image description, including left ventricular size, ejection fraction, and wall motion abnormalities, if present; (h) any other pertinent notes.

The editors encourage readers and nuclear cardiology practitioners to not delay reporting and to try to send a signed report within one day of the test. This will enhance patient care and lead to appropriate management decisions. Prompt and clear reporting is indeed a quality measure of any nuclear cardiology practice.

Noncardiac Findings in SPECT

Noncardiac findings have been described in many studies.[23] It should be kept in mind that cardiac SPECT uses tracers that are also used for the diagnosis of tumors, and if there is any suspicious uptake it should be included in the report and communicated directly to the referring physician. One of the most common sources of noncardiac findings is contaminants. They are usually present in only one set of images (rest or stress), since they are often detected and removed by the technologist, and they tend to be superficial since they are on the skin. On the other hand, tumor activities are typically present in both sets of images, with higher clarity in the high dose images (usually the stress images). Tumor activities tend to be deeper and localized to certain organs such as lungs or breasts.

Following is a case that demonstrates the importance of paying attention to extra-cardiac findings:

A 79-year-old man with cardiac risk factor of hypercholesteremia and hypertension presented for evaluation of exertional chest pain. He underwent Tc-99m sestambi treadmill stress test.

Results of myocardial perfusion scan are shown in Figure 2.15.

The myocardial perfusion scans revealed inferior ischemia, and the raw data (Figure 2.16) showed a spot of extra-cardiac activity (arrow in figure). The ordering physician was contacted and a CT scan showed a rounded mass in the left breast 2.8 cm in diameter, raising concern for a malignancy (Figure 2.17).

The patient underwent modified radical mastectomy with pathology revealing invasive cell carcinoma. The patient also had cardiac catheterization that showed totally occluded mid right coronary artery (RCA) with collaterals from obtuse marginal with 90% stenosis, which was successfully stented.

The case above is an example of the importance of noting noncardiac uptakes on the raw data (rotatograms) and reporting them. However, it should be kept in mind that these findings are very rare, especially with newer cameras, which have a smaller field of view that concentrates mainly on the heart.

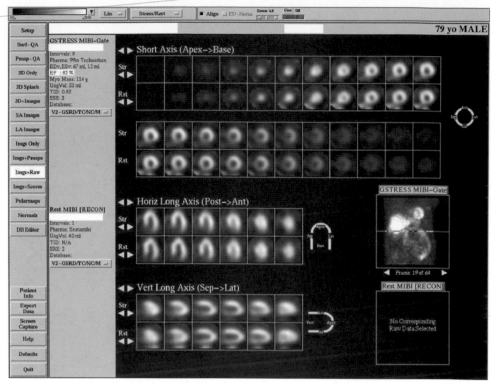

FIGURE 2.15   Myocardial perfusion scan.

FIGURE 2.16   Rotatogram (raw data) with extra cardiac tracer uptake (arrow).

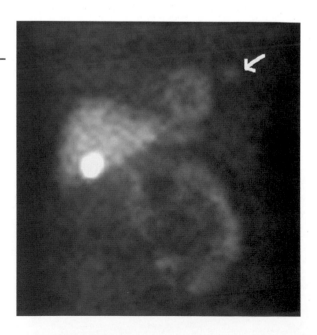

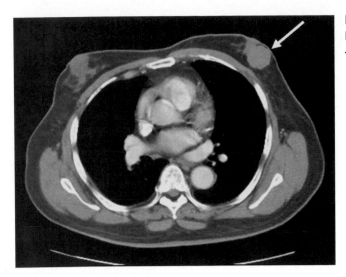

FIGURE 2.17   CT scan with mass in left breast area (arrow).

SPECT Viability Studies

Although fluorodeoxyglucose–positron emission tomography (FDG-PET) scans are considered the gold standard for cardiac viability, SPECT studies are still very commonly used for that pupose because of the availability of the technology and good accuracy. There are many protocols, the most common being Thallium based. These protocols are based on the fact that Thallium is an element very close to potassium, and Thallium redistributes to living (hibernating or viable) cells that get low perfusion in the early set of imaging and appear to be infarcted. Many Thallium protocols have been proposed and used and are shown in Figure 2.18. It has also been proposed that sestamibi can be used as a viability tracer with protocols involving the use of nitroglycerin to enhance myocardial uptake.[22,23]

FIGURE 2.18   Thallium viability protocols.

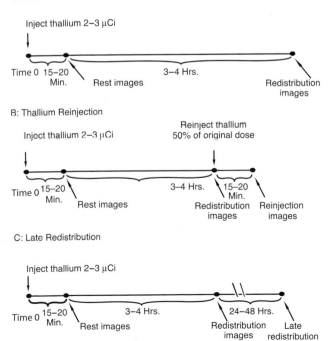

CT/SPECT

CT/SPECT is performed using a hybrid nuclear camera and a CT machine. The CT part can be used to perform attenuation correction. Also, the CT can be used to perform coronary CT angiography that will give important anatomic information in addition to the physiologic data of the myocardial perfusion scan. However, hybrid machines that include a 64-slice CT are not available commercially yet, and it appears that the CT/PET arena is progressing at a faster pace, as discussed in a different chapter.

Office-Based Nuclear Cardiology

As a result of the recent advances in nuclear cameras that have made them smaller and more efficient, the practice of office-based nuclear cardiology has expanded tremendously. All major companies have produced small and efficient cameras that can be fitted in a small office space. Examples of these cameras include the c.cam from Siemens, the CardioMD by Phillips, the Cardius camera by Digirad, and the Ventri by GE.

Setting Up an Office-Based Nuclear Cardiology Lab

In order to obtain a license to perform nuclear cardiology studies from the Nuclear Regulatory Commission (NRC), the practice must fulfill many requirements. Below are some of these requirements:

1. Supplying a business name and address.
2. Becoming an authorized user with training qualifications accepted by the NRC.
3. Having a radiation safety officer (RSO) with training qualifications accepted by the NRC.
4. Supplying the business license for the facility.
5. Identification of the nuclear camera to be used with the name of the company and model number.
6. Specifying the requested isotope and activity that will be required.
7. Submitting an overall facility diagram, including adjacent buildings and parking areas. This should include prep areas, injection areas, patient waiting rooms, treadmill location, and imaging rooms.
8. Submitting an enlarged, labeled hot lab diagram, including use, storage, and waste areas.
9. Description of how security is maintained in the building.
10. Description of all isotope use and storage areas.
11. Description of personnel training program.
12. Description of all the daily surveys completed at the end of the day.
13. Building owner agreement.

Radiation Safety Officer Duties and Responsibilities

It is an absolute requirement for the licensing of any nuclear cardiology practice to have a qualified radiation safety officer to oversee the use of radioactive isotopes and ensure the compliance of the practice to all NRC and state regulations. Depending on their qualifications and training, an authorized user can be the RSO or the role can be assigned to a different person who fulfills the requirement.

RSO duties and responsibilities include ensuring radiological safety and compliance with the State, U.S. NRC, and Department of Transportation (DOT) regulations and the conditions of the license. These duties and responsibilities include ensuring that

• Radiation exposures are ALARA.
• 10 CFR Part 20 and investigational levels are followed.

- Radiation protection procedures in the daily operation of the licensee's radioactive material programs are developed, distributed, implemented, and up to date.
- Possession, use, and storage of licensed material are consistent with the limitations in the license, the regulations, the National Sealed Source and Device Registry (NSSDR) certificate(s), and the manufacturer's recommendations and instructions.
- Individuals installing, relocating, maintaining, or repairing devices containing sealed sources are trained and authorized by an NRC or an Agreement State license.
- Training of personnel is conducted and is commensurate with the individual's duties regarding licensed material.
- Any activity involving licensed material that the RSO considers unsafe is stopped.
- Determination that individuals are not likely to receive, in one year, a radiation dose in excess of 10% of the allowable limits.
- Documentation as to the issuance of dosimetry if an individual(s) is determined to be likely to receive, in one year, a radiation dose in excess of 10% of the allowable limits.
- When necessary, [personnel] monitoring devices are used and exchanged at the proper intervals, and records of the results of such monitoring are maintained.
- Licensed material is properly secured.
- The RSO is to verify that the total effective dose equivalent does not exceed the annual limit for members of the public. This determination is to be documented by measurement or calculation.
- Proper authorities are notified of incidents such as loss or theft of licensed material, damage to or malfunction of sealed sources, and fire.
- Medical events are investigated and reported to the State Department of Public Health, Radiologic Health Branch, as specified in title 10, Code of Federal Regulations, Part 35, section 35.2 and section 35.3045.
- Audits of the radiation protection programs are performed and documented at least annually.
- Violations of regulations or license conditions, or program weaknesses, are identified and effective corrective actions are developed, implemented, and documented, as needed.
- Licensed material is transported in accordance with all applicable DOT requirements.
- Licensed material is properly disposed of.
- Appropriate records are maintained.

Intersocietal Commission for the Accreditation of Nuclear Medicine Laboratories Certification

The Intersocietal Commission for the Accreditation of Nuclear Medicine Laboratories (ICANL) is dedicated to promoting quality nuclear cardiology and nuclear medicine diagnostic evaluations in the delivery of health care by providing a peer review process of laboratory accreditation. The ICANL sponsored by the Academy of Molecular Imaging, American College of Cardiology, American College of Nuclear Physicians, American Society of Nuclear Cardiology, and the Society of Nuclear Medicine. It sets the standards for the accreditation of nuclear cardiology facilities and for different aspects of nuclear cardiology facilities, including the medical director, the medical staff, nuclear medicine technologists, equipment and documentation, procedures and protocols, and quality improvement measures. Further details of these standards are published on the ICANL Web site (see Appendix 1).

The editors of this book strongly encourage pursuing ICANL certification since it will enhance the quality of patient care. In addition, some private insurance companies have started requiring this certification as a condition for paying for services provided by nuclear cardiology practices.

TABLE 2-17	Common Billing Codes for Office Based Nuclear Cardiology
78465	SPECT S/R myocardial perfusion
78478	Myocardial perfusion with wall motion
78480	Myocardial perfusion with EF
93015	Cardiovascular stress test
A9500	Cardiolite up to 40 mCi # units _____ (rest dose)
A9500	Cardiolite up to 40 mCi # units _____ (stress dose)
J1245	Persantine up to 10 mg # units _____
J0152	Adenosine up to 30 mg # units _____
J7050	Normal saline 250 cc

Commonly Used Billing Codes in Office-Based Nuclear Cardiology

Table 2.17 shows some of the commonly used billing codes in office-based nuclear cardiology. For the details of each of these codes and for other codes that involve different tracers or different types of tests, please refer to the latest edition of the Current Procedural Terminology (CPT) manual.

The Certification Board of Nuclear Cardiology

The information below was obtained from the Certification Board of Nuclear Cardiology (CBNC) Web site (see Appendix 1). The editors of this book strongly recommend pursuing CBNC certification since it will enhance the appropriate practice of nuclear cardiology and will facilitate licensing by the NRC board.

Mission

The mission of the Certification Board of Nuclear Cardiology (CBNC) is to support optimal patient care and enhancement of the field through a certification program that promotes quality, professionalism, and practice-based learning and improvement.

The Certification Board of Nuclear Cardiology (CBNC) is committed to the certification of Nuclear Cardiology practitioners. Certification will provide practice-based requirements against which members of the profession can be assessed. The purposes of the CBNC Certification Program are as follows:

- to establish the domain of the practice of Nuclear Cardiology for certification;
- to assess the level of knowledge demonstrated by Nuclear Cardiology specialists in a valid manner;
- to encourage professional growth in, and enhance the quality of, the practice of Nuclear Cardiology;
- to recognize formally individuals who meet the requirements set by CBNC; and
- to serve the public by encouraging quality patient care in the practice of Nuclear Cardiology.

Eligibility
2007 Certification Eligibility Requirements for Candidates Residing in the United States
Requirement 1: Licensure
Applicants must, at the time of application, hold a current, unconditional, unrestricted license to practice medicine in the U.S. and must provide a copy of the current license.

Requirement 2: Board Certification

Applicants must be physicians who, at the time of application, are Board Certified in Cardiology, Nuclear Medicine, or Radiology by a board which holds membership in either the American Board of Medical Specialties, or the Bureau of Osteopathic Specialists of the American Osteopathic Association.

Applicants with Internal Medicine Board Certification may apply but will not receive a certificate upon successful completion of the exam until they provide documentation of successful certification in Cardiology, Nuclear Medicine or Radiology, which must happen within 2 years of sitting for the CBNC exam. Assuming this happens, the certification period will be 10 years from the date of the successful nuclear cardiology exam.

Requirement 3: Training/Experience in the Provision of Nuclear Cardiology Services (Training Must Be Complete Prior to Application)

Pathway 1—For candidates who received nuclear cardiology training during an ACGME-accredited residency or fellowship program in Cardiovascular Disease, Nuclear Medicine, or Radiology, 1998 or later. Nuclear cardiology training must have met the ACCF/ASNC COCATS Guidelines for Training in Nuclear Cardiology, Revised 2006, for a minimum of Level 2 training (see Appendix 2). A preceptor letter must be provided.

A preceptor must be one of the following:

- Program Director of an accredited residency or fellowship program in Cardiovascular Disease, Nuclear Medicine, or Radiology.
- Director of Nuclear Cardiology laboratory at an institution with an accredited residency or fellowship program in Cardiovascular Disease, Nuclear Medicine, or Radiology.

If the preceptor is not an Authorized User, a separate letter from an Authorized User must be provided to verify that the candidate has had appropriate training in radiation safety.

The preceptor letter must be dated no earlier than 12 months prior to application and must document the training dates of the applicant.

Candidates must provide separate documentation that they are either an Authorized User *(e.g., copy of current facility radioactive materials license listing the applicant's name)* or eligible to become an Authorized User *(e.g., a certificate of completion of a course with a minimum of 80 hours which included ALL the topic areas required by the Nuclear Regulatory Commission OR a statement from the applicant's preceptor if the hours were taken directly within the fellowship program. See language below).*

Pathway 2—For candidates trained before 1998, OR candidates who trained after 1998 but who did not receive nuclear cardiology training within the context of an accredited residency or fellowship program. Nuclear cardiology training and/or experience must have met the ACCF/ASNC COCATS Guidelines for Training in Nuclear Cardiology, Revised 2006, for a minimum of Level 2 training equivalent. These candidates must document:

1. Authorized User status *(e.g., copy of current facility radioactive materials license listing the applicant's name)* or Authorized User eligibility *(e.g., a certificate of completion of a course with a minimum of 80 hours which included ALL topic areas required by the Nuclear Regulatory Commission).*
2. Ongoing experience as evidenced by interpretation of a minimum of 300 cases (current Nuclear Cardiology COCATS requirement for Level 2) in the preceding 2 years; letter templates available at the CBNC Web site.
3. At least 25 hours of CME specific to nuclear cardiology within the preceding 3 years.

A preceptor letter must be provided. The preceptor must be certified by one of the following Boards: CBNC, ABNM, ABR, AOBNM, or AOBR. ABIM certification alone does NOT qualify.

If the preceptor is not an Authorized User, a separate letter from an Authorized User must be provided to verify that the candidate has had appropriate training in radiation safety.

The preceptor letter must be dated no earlier than 12 months prior to application and must document the training dates of the applicant.

> **NOTE:** All U.S. Candidates must submit evidence of either Authorized User status *(e.g., a copy of the facility's radioactive materials license listing the Candidate's name)*, OR of Authorized User eligibility *(e.g., a certificate of completion of a radioisotope handling and radiation safety course with a minimum of 80 hours which included ALL topic areas required by the Nuclear Regulatory Commission and dated within 7 years of application)*.
>
> If the Classroom and Laboratory Training hours were a direct part of the fellowship program, the candidate's preceptor should include the following text in his/her preceptor attestation:
>
> **Dr. _____ completed XX hours of Radioisotope Handling Classroom and Laboratory Training which meets the requirements of the Nuclear Regulatory Commission within his/her fellowship program.**

NOTE: The preceptor verifying training/experience must include in the preceptor letter his or her NRC or Agreement State License Number.

Training and experience requirements for licensure by the Nuclear Regulatory Commission (NRC) or Agreement States vary from state to state; therefore, Candidates seeking licensure should check with their regional NRC office or the office responsible for licensure in the Agreement State in which they practice. Information is also available on the NRC Web site (see Appendix 1).

New in 2007

- Preceptor letters must be sent directly from the preceptor to the CBNC office. Preceptor letters which accompany the application will be returned to the candidate for noncompliance. Preceptor templates may be found on the CBNC Web site.
- Preceptor letters must be dated no earlier than 12 months prior to application.
- Preceptor letters must be on organizational letterhead and the author's relationship to the applicant provided (e.g., Program Director).
- The letter must include the applicant's training dates.
- If the preceptor is not an Authorized User, a separate letter from an Authorized User must be provided to verify that the candidate has had appropriate training in radiation safety.

2007 Eligibility Requirements for Candidates Residing Outside the United States or with Training from Outside the United States

> **NOTE: Candidates who meet any criteria from outside the U.S. will receive a non-U.S. certificate when they pass the exam. These certificates are not transferable to U.S.-certificates at any time. If an individual relocates to the U.S., and subsequently satisfies all requirements for a U.S. candidate, he/she must retake the examination to obtain a U.S. certificate.**

Requirement 1: Licensure
Applicants must, at the time of application, hold a current, unconditional, unrestricted license to practice medicine and must provide a copy of the current license.

Requirement 2: Training/Experience in the Provision of Nuclear Cardiology Services (Must Be Complete at the Time of Application)

Pathway 1—For applicants who have completed training in cardiology, nuclear medicine, or radiology after July 1, 1998, you must submit a statement written on organizational letterhead, within the last 12 months, from your preceptor stating that your training in nuclear cardiology was equivalent to ACCF/ASNC COCATS Guidelines for Nuclear Cardiology Training, Revised 2006, Level 2 (minimum). Your preceptor may be:

- Program Director of a residency or fellowship in Cardiovascular Disease, Nuclear Medicine, or Radiology
- Director of Nuclear Cardiology laboratory at an institution with a residency or fellowship in Cardiovascular Disease, Nuclear Medicine, or Radiology

Pathway 2—For applicants who have completed training in cardiology, nuclear medicine, or radiology prior to July 1, 1998, you must submit a statement from a preceptor, written on organizational letterhead within the last 12 months, that verifies ongoing experience as evidenced by interpretation of a minimum of 300 cases per year (current Nuclear Cardiology COCATS requirement for Level 2 training) in the preceding 2 years.

A preceptor letter must be provided (template can be obtained from CBNC Web site).

Examination Content Outline (Revised 2006)

Following is a detailed outline of the nine major content areas of the examination, with an indication (in parentheses) of the approximate percentage of the examination devoted to each area:

I. PHYSICS AND INSTRUMENTATION (10%) (5% in Recertification Examination)
   A. Basic physics as applied to clinical imaging (e.g., isotope decay, decay modes, generators, high energy imaging)
   B. Gamma cameras, collimation, and equipment quality control procedures
   C. Interactions of radiation with matter
   D. Attenuation correction, including transmission and CT methods

II. RADIOPHARMACEUTICALS (8%)
   A. Radiotracer kinetics and characteristics (e.g., Thallium-201 and technetium-99m)
   B. PET agents
   C. Red blood cell tagging

III. RADIATION SAFETY (10%) (15% in Recertification Examination)
   A. Radiopharmaceutical receiving, handling, monitoring, and containment
   B. Handling radiopharmaceutical spills and waste
   C. Storage and calibration of radiopharmaceuticals
   D. Dosimetry and MIRD
   E. Radiation exposure and ALARA
   F. Governmental regulations

IV. NUCLEAR CARDIOLOGY DIAGNOSTIC TESTS AND PROCEDURES/ PROTOCOLS (15%)
   A. Image acquisition (e.g., first pass and equilibrium RNA, gating, SPECT)
   B. Image processing (e.g., filtering, reorientation, reconstruction, motion correction)
   C. Standard conventions as to how images are displayed
   D. Exercise and pharmacologic stress protocols
   E. Pharmacologic stress agents

F. Artifacts and causes of false-positive and false-negative results

G. Quality control of image processing

H. Quality assurance of interpretation

I. Quantitative aids to interpretation

V. GENERAL CARDIOLOGY AS IT RELATES TO IMAGE INTERPRETATION (10%)

A. Coronary anatomy and pathophysiology

B. Unique characteristics of patient subgroups (e.g., patients with diabetes, elderly patients, male vs. female patients)

C. Coronary angiography

D. Stress physiology and testing; ECG and clinical parameters with rest and stress

E. Measurements of left ventricle systolic and diastolic function

F. Valvular disease, cardiomyopathy, hypertension, CHF, myocarditis

G. Endothelial dysfunction

H. Coronary artery disease

I. Medical therapy, percutaneous coronary intervention, and coronary bypass surgery

J. Indications for the use of alternative diagnostic techniques (echo, MRI, coronary calcification, CT angiography)

K. Bayes' theorem, pre- and post-test likelihood, sensitivity, specificity, and referral bias

L. Statistical analyses (e.g., kappa value, Bland-Altman, ROC curves, Kaplan-Meier)

M. Cost-effectiveness of diagnostic tests and principles of outcome studies

VI. RISK STRATIFICATION (10%)

A. Coronary artery disease

B. Unstable angina

C. Acute myocardial infarction

D. Acute chest pain

E. Candidates for noncardiac surgery

F. Diabetes

G. Chronic renal disease

H. Women

I. Post revascularization: percutaneous coronary intervention and CABG

J. Evaluation of medical therapy

VII. MYOCARDIAL PERFUSION IMAGING INTERPRETATION (22%)

A. Interpretation of perfusion images with technetium-99m-labeled tracers and Thallium-201

B. Interpretation of images with rubidium-82 and N-13-ammonia

C. Relationship of perfusion abnormalities to clinical, hemodynamic, ECG, and exercise parameters

D. Relationship of perfusion abnormalities to coronary anatomy

E. Combined function-perfusion imaging

VIII. VENTRICULAR FUNCTION IMAGING (10%)

A. Rest and stress first-pass radionuclide ventriculography

B. Rest and rest/stress equilibrium radionuclide ventriculography (planar and SPECT), including volume measurements and systolic and diastolic function

C. ECG-gated SPECT myocardial perfusion imaging

D. Effect of arrhythmia on ECG gating

E. Implications of ventricular function testing for clinical management

IX. MYOCARDIAL VIABILITY (5%)

A. Thallium-201 imaging

B. Technetium-99m imaging

C. FDG imaging

D. Outcome data related to myocardial viability

E. Relationship to other imaging methods (e.g., echo, MRI)

REFERENCES

1. Brindis RG, Douglas PS, Hendel RC, et al. ACCF/ASNC appropriateness criteria for single-photon emission computed tomography myocardial perfusion imaging (SPECT MPI): A report of the American College of Cardiology Foundation Quality Strategic Directions Committee Appropriateness Criteria Working Group and the American Society of Nuclear Cardiology endorsed by the American Heart Association. *J Am Coll Cardiol.* 2005; 46:1587–1605.

2. Hachamovitch R, Berman DS, Kiat H, et al. Incremental prognostic value of Adenosine stress myocardial perfusion single-photon emission computed tomography and impact on subsequent management in patients with or suspected of having myocardial ischemia. *Am J Cardiol.* 1997; 80:426–433.

3. Basu S, Senior R, Dore C, Lahiri A. Value of Thallium-201 imaging in detecting adverse cardiac events after myocardial infarction and thrombolysis: A follow up of 100 consecutive patients. *BMJ.* 1996; 313:844–848.

4. Brown KA, Heller GV, Landin RS, et al. Early dipyridamole (99m)Tc-sestamibi single photon emission computed tomographic imaging 2 to 4 days after acute myocardial infarction predicts in-hospital and postdischarge cardiac events: comparison with submaximal exercise imaging. *Circulation.* 1999; 100:2060–2066.

5. Dakik HA, Mahmarian JJ, Kimball KT, Koutelou MG, Medrano R, Verani MS. Prognostic value of exercise 201Tl tomography in patients treated with thrombolytic therapy during acute myocardial infarction. *Circulation.* 1996; 94:2735–2742.

6. Verani MS. Risk stratifying patients who survive an acute myocardial infarction. *J Nucl Cardiol.* 1998; 5:96–108.

7. Hachamovitch R, Hayes SW, Friedman JD, Cohen I, Berman DS. Comparison of the short-term survival benefit associated with revascularization compared with medical therapy in patients with no prior coronary artery disease undergoing stress myocardial perfusion single photon emission computed tomography. *Circulation.* 2003; 107:2900–2907.

8. Gibbons RJ, Balady GJ, Bricker JT, et al. ACC/AHA 2002 guideline update for exercise testing: Summary article. A report of the American College of Cardiology/American Heart Association Task Force on Practice Guidelines (Committee to Update the 1997 Exercise Testing Guidelines). *J Am Coll Cardiol.* 2002; 40:1531–1540.

9. Ami E. Iskandrian, MD, FACC, Timothy M. Bateman, MD, FACC, Luiz Belardinelli, MD, Brent Blackburn, PhD, Manual D. Cerqueira, MD, FACC, Robert C. Hendel, MD, FACC, Ann Olmsted, PhD, S. Richard Underwood, MD. FACC, joao Vitola, MD, and Whedy Wang, PhD, on behalf of the ADVANCE MPI Investigators

10. Sharir T, Germano G, Kang X, et al. Prediction of myocardial infarction versus cardiac death by gated myocardial perfusion SPECT: Risk stratification by the amount of stress-induced ischemia and the poststress ejection fraction. *J Nucl Med.* 2001; 42:831–837.

11. Ficaro EP, Fessler JA, Shreve PD, Kritzman JN, Rose PA, Corbett JR. Simultaneous transmission/emission myocardial perfusion tomography. Diagnostic accuracy of attenuation-corrected 99mTc-sestamibi single-photon emission computed tomography. *Circulation.* 1996; 93:463–473.

12. Ficaro EP, Fessler JA, Ackermann RJ, Rogers WL, Corbett JR, Schwaiger M. Simultaneous transmission-emission Thallium-201 cardiac SPECT: Effect of attenuation correction on myocardial tracer distribution. *J Nucl Med.* 1995; 36:921–931.

13. Kluge R, Sattler B, Seese A, Knapp WH. Attenuation correction by simultaneous emission-transmission myocardial single-photon emission tomography using a technetium-99m-labelled radiotracer: Impact on diagnostic accuracy. *Eur J Nucl Med.* 1997; 24:1107–1114.

14. Gallowitsch HJ, Sykora J, Mikosch P, et al. Attenuation-corrected Thallium-201 single-photon emission tomography using a gadolinium-153 moving line source: clinical value and the impact of attenuation correction on the extent and severity of perfusion abnormalities. *Eur J Nucl Med.* 1998; 25:220–228.

15. Leslie WD, Yogendran MS, Ward LM, Nour KA, Metge CJ. Prognostic utility of sestamibi lung uptake does not require adjustment for stress-related variables: A retrospective cohort study. *BMC Nucl Med.* 2006; 6:2.

16. Klocke FJ, Baird MG, Lorell BH, et al. ACC/AHA/ASNC guidelines for the clinical use of cardiac radionuclide imaging—executive summary: A report of the American College of Cardiology/American Heart Association Task Force on Practice Guidelines (ACC/AHA/ASNC Committee to Revise the 1995 Guidelines for the Clinical Use of Cardiac Radionuclide Imaging). *J Am Coll Cardiol.* 2003; 42:1318–1333.

17. Scott JA. Using artificial neural network analysis of global ventilation-perfusion scan morphometry as a diagnostic tool. *AJR Am J Roentgenol*. 1999; 173:943–948.

18. Scott JA, Palmer EL, Fischman AJ. How well can radiologists using neural network software diagnose pulmonary embolism? *AJR Am J Roentgenol*. 2000; 175:399–405.

19. Scott JA, Aziz K, Yasuda T, Gewirtz H. Integration of clinical and imaging data to predict the presence of coronary artery disease with the use of neural networks. *Coron Artery Dis*. 2004; 15:427–434.

20. Lim MJ, Kern MJ. Coronary pathophysiology in the cardiac catheterization laboratory. *Curr Probl Cardiol*. 2006; 31:493–550.

21. Jones SE, Aziz K, Yasuda T, et al. To test the hypothessis that the observed incidence of important noncardiac findings (NCFs) on myocardial perfusion imaging increases. *Nucl Med Commun*. 2008; 29(7):607–613.

22. Giorgetti A, Pingitore A, Favilli B, Kusch A, Lombardi M, Marzullo P. Baseline/postnitrate tetrofosmin SPECT for myocardial viability assessment in patients with postischemic severe left ventricular dysfunction: new evidence from MRI. *J Nucl Med*. 2005; 46:1285–1293.

23. Tzonevska A, Tzvetkov K, Dimitrova M, Piperkova E. Assessment of myocardial viability with (99m)Tc-sestamibi-gated SPET images in patients undergoing percutaneous transluminar coronary angioplasty. *Hell J Nucl Med*. 2005; 8:48–53.

CHAPTER 3

Kusai S. Aziz

Equilibrium Radionuclide Angiography

Current Uses and Protocols

The other name for equilibrium radionuclide angiography (ERNA) is MUGA (multi-gated acquisition) scans. It is used mainly for evaluation of left ventricular systolic function at rest. However, ERNA can also be used for other indications such as evaluation of right ventricular systolic function or for the diagnosis of coronary artery disease when it is combined with exercise by looking for post exercise drop of left ventricular ejection fraction (LVEF). The use of this technique has declined during the last several years because of the widespread use of less time-consuming tests to evaluate systolic function, such as echocardiogram, and because of the introduction of gating in single photon emission computed tomography (SPECT) myocardial perfusion imaging, which calculates left ventricular ejection fraction and gives an idea about wall motion. However, it should kept in mind that MUGA scans are the most accurate and reproducible technique for EF calculation since they depend on the count numbers during systole and diastole, and unlike echocardiogram or gated SPECT do not have geometric assumptions that can lead to false LVEF calculations. Therefore, these scans still used when accurate evaluation of LVEF is needed, and as a tie-breaker when there are conflicting measurements of LVEF.

Technetium-99m labeled red blood cells (RBCs) are most commonly used in this technique. The RBCs can be labeled in vivo by injecting tracer (sodium pertechnetate) after stannous pyrophosphate, or more commonly in vitro by removing 50 mL of blood in a syringe and adding stannous pyrophosphate followed by the radioactive sodium pertechnetate. The stannous pyrophosphate function is to attach (glue) the radioactive sodium pertechnetate to the RBCs. Finally, there is the combined in vitro and in vivo technique (in vivtro) in which 50 mL of blood is removed in a syringe, mixed with stannous pyrophosphate, and injected back into the patient. This is followed by injection of the radioactive sodium pertechnetate.[1]

Layouts and Definitions

Planar gated images are then acquired in anterior and lateral anterior oblique views (Figures 3.1 and 3.2). The user uses software to measure activity at end diastole and end systole and the ejection fraction is calculated using the following formula:

$$EF = (\text{end diastolic counts} - \text{end systolic counts})/\text{end diastolic counts}$$

The software is usually used to subtract background activity. It should be kept in mind that ERNA can be helpful in diagnosing abnormalities in other cardiac chambers such as right ventricular enlargement (Figure 3.3).

FIGURE 3.1 Views of equilibrium radionuclide angiography (ERNA) (multi-gated acquisition [MUGA]) scan.

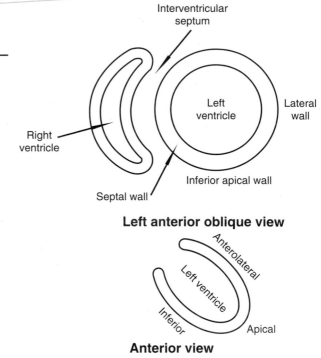

Sources of Errors

There are many sources of errors in this technique, including patient motion artifacts, low hematocrit, and medications such as heparin, digoxin, and hydralazine.[2] Another common source of error is high background activity, which can falsely elevate EF since it is subtracted from both end systolic and end diastolic counts.

FIGURE 3.2 Correct positioning of left ventricle.
Reproduced with permission from DePuey EG. Evaluation of cardiac function with radionuclides. In: Gottschalk A, Hoffer PB, Potchen EJ, eds. *Diagnostic Nuclear Medicine.* Baltimore: Williams and Wilkins; 1998.

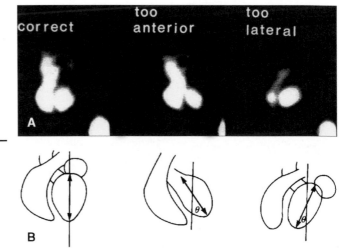

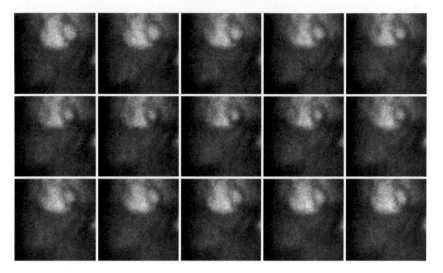

FIGURE 3.3 Equilibrium radionuclide angiography (ERNA) scan showing severe right ventricular enlargement compared to small size left ventricle.

REFERENCES

1. Klocke FJ, Baird MG, Lorell BH, et al. ACC/AHA/ASNC guidelines for the clinical use of cardiac radionuclide imaging—executive summary: A report of the American College of Cardiology/American Heart Association Task Force on Practice Guidelines (ACC/AHA/ASNC Committee to Revise the 1995 Guidelines for the Clinical Use of Cardiac Radionuclide Imaging). *J Am Coll Cardiol. 2003* Oct 1; 42(7):1318–1333.
2. Port SC, Berman D, Garcia EG. Imaging guidelines for nuclear cardiology procedures—part 2. *J Nucl Cardiol.* 1999; 6:G47–G84.

Cardiac Positron Emission Tomography (PET)

4.1   Basic PET Physics and the PET Camera

Kusai S. Aziz

As mentioned earlier, some radionuclides decay by positron emission; a positively charged electron is emitted from the nucleus, and after travelling a few millimeters it interacts with an electron in an annihilation reaction that leads to the production of two high energy photons (511 MeV) at 180° to each other (Figure 4.1). The PET camera is built based on the unique characteristics of these photons. The camera is supplied by scintillating crystals at 360° and a coincident circuit is used to detect these photons that hit the camera at 180° at the same time. These photons will be considered in constructing the nuclear scans, and other photons that do not meet these criteria will be considered scattered photons and will be ignored (Figure 4.2). The PET camera scintillating crystals are different from those used for single photon emission computed tomography (SPECT) cameras, and they are usually made of $Bi_4Ge_3O_{12}$ (bismuth germanate, or BGO). The smaller the crystals are, the higher the resolution of that PET camera. The crystals are connected to a photomultiplier tube that converts the light signal into an electrical one.

FIGURE 4.1   Positron emission.

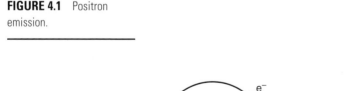
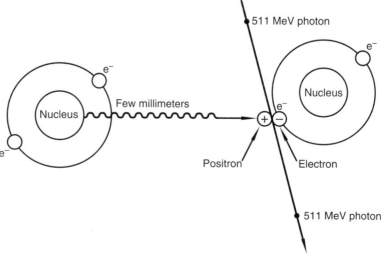

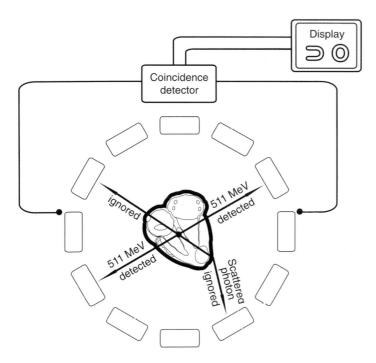

FIGURE 4.2 Basic structure of a positron emission tomography (PET) camera.

Because of the above factors, cardiac PET results have more resolution than cardiac SPECT and are more accurate. PET scans require an initial scan called a transmission scan, which is performed using a rotating radioactive source built into the machine for attenuation correction, or it can be done through low energy computed tomography (CT) radiation in the case of combined CT/PET machines. Following this the emission scan is performed to track the injected nuclear tracer. Every effort should be made to avoid patient movement between the two scans since the misregistration of these two sets of scans could be a source of false results. One solution to such a problem is to repeat the transmission scans after the emission scans.

4.2   PET Tracers

Kusai S. Aziz

F-18 FDG (F-18 fluorodeoxyglucose)

- Myocardial metabolic tracer.
- Main PET tracer in cardiology and oncology.
- Half-life 110 minutes.
- Cyclotron produced.
- Used mainly for viability studies.
- More details are discussed in the myocardial viability chapter.

N-13 ammonia

- Myocardial perfusion tracer
- Excellent image quality
- Good high flow correlation, therefore good quantitative blood flow
- Halflife 10 minutes
- Cyclotron produced

Rubidium-82 (Rb82)

- Myocardial perfusion agent.
- Half-life 76 seconds.
- Generator connected to the patient.
- Can give up to 50 μCi per dose.
- Similar to K and Thallium, but cannot be used as viability agent because of short half-life.
- Poor quantitative agent because poor correlation with high blood flow.
- Rb 82 is generator produced.

O-15 water

- Cyclotron produced.
- Half-life 110 seconds (biggest limitation).
- Used mainly for research.
- Best quantitative agent.
- Relation to blood flow is linear because of free diffusion of water.

C-11 palmitate

- Cyclotron produced
- Half-life 20 minutes
- Fatty acid, used historically as a viability agent

Technetium (Tc) tracers

- Tc has 33 isotopes, from ^{85}Tc to ^{117}Tc.
- Many of them are positron emitters.
- High resolution positrons.

C-11 acetate

- Cyclotron produced
- Half-life 20 minutes
- Good correlation with high blood flow
- Used for research only in a few centers
- Enters acetic acid cycle
- Is used as flow agent, and is the *only* tracer to measure myocardial oxygen consumption
- Potential for very early detection of heart disease

4.3   PET Measurement of Myocardial Blood Flow

Henry Gewirtz

Introduction

The use of PET as a method for measuring myocardial blood flow (MBF) dates to the pioneering work of Schelbert, Gould, Bergmann, and Sobel in the late 1970s and early 1980s.[1-3] The most commonly employed radiotracers used for this purpose have been O-15 water, N-13 ammonia, and rubidium-82.[4,5] Initial efforts at making the technology clinically relevant were hampered by the need for an on-site cyclotron and associated infrastructure to produce the radionuclides. Accordingly, PET for measurement of myocardial blood flow (and metabolism) was largely confined to a few experimental laboratories in the United States and Europe.

The more recent commercialization and proliferation of PET scanners has been driven by the discovery that [18]fluorodeoxyglucose (FDG), a relatively long-lived positron emitter (T 1/2 ~ 2 hours), is a tumor avid agent and so has been found to be helpful in the management of patients with many types of cancer.[6-8] The 2-hour half-life of the isotope also meant that an on-site cyclotron was unnecessary since the tracer could be ordered from relatively nearby commercial facilities and shipped to hospitals and outpatient imaging centers equipped with PET scanners.

The development of a generator/delivery system for rubidium-82[9] has obviated the need for a cyclotron to produce an MBF tracer and, along with the proliferation of PET oncology, has fueled a substantial increase in PET myocardial perfusion studies. Accordingly, the technology has moved from being strictly a research tool requiring a substantial infrastructure of both human and material resources to a clinically applicable tool that is enjoying more widespread use all the time. As such, it behooves the cardiologist-in-training to be familiar with the technique and its major applications, as well as its strengths and weaknesses.

Methodologies

Positron Imaging

PET imaging differs fundamentally from standard SPECT in the following ways: The radiotracers employed for PET imaging are positron emitters, which move only a short distance in tissue (~1–4 mm) after which they encounter a negative electron (Figure 4.3). The encounter results in annihilation of both particles and the release of two 511 keV photons at 180° angles from one another. The 511 keV photons can be recognized by special detectors, commonly bismuth germanium oxide (BGO), housed in a gantry resembling that of a CT scanner, which surrounds the patient. Details of the mathematics and electronics required for image reconstruction are beyond the scope of this review. It is important, however, to point out that since two photons are involved for each annihilation event, it is possible to accurately position where the event took place (within the 1–4 mm distance the particle migrated prior to annihilation) and the number of true, as opposed to random (i.e., unpaired) events that occurred. Then, using a transmission scan of the patient typically obtained prior to injection of any radioactivity, it is possible to accurately correct for photon attenuation, which occurs as the 511 keV photons exit the body, and thereby determine with considerable accuracy not only where the events took place but how many there were (i.e., the quantity of tracer present in a given location at a given moment in time). The data are then fit to a tracer kinetic model (see below), which is used to define absolute myocardial blood flow (or metabolic parameters depending on tracer employed) in quantitative terms (Figures 4.4A and B).

FIGURE 4.3 An illustration of a greatly simplified PET scanner is shown here. A positron (*circle with plus*) encounters an electron (*circle with minus*) and an annihilation event occurs with two 511 keV photons traveling away from one another at a 180° angle. Since both are in the field of view of the opposed detectors, the event is counted and can be accurately localized. Other events occurring outside the field of view of the two detectors are not recognized in this simplified example. PET, positron emission tomography.

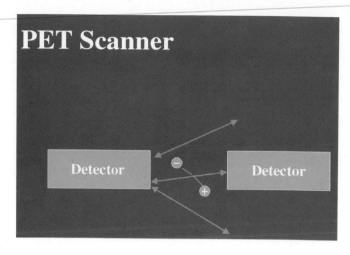

FIGURE 4.4 See color figure on website. (*A*) An illustration of a tracer kinetic model for MBF is shown here. The parameter K1 reflects MBF in mL/min/g. The terms k2 and k3 reflect back diffusion of the tracer into the blood and incorporation of the N-13 label into glutamine, respectively. (*B*) Time activity curves for left ventricle (*red*) and myocardium (*blue*) are shown here. The dotted lines represent the fit of the data to the tracer kinetic model shown schematically in Figure 4.4A. Note the robust fit of the data to the model ($r^2 = 0.94$). The value of K1 (0.84) reflects MBF in mL/min/g but requires correction for incomplete extraction of the tracer (see text for details). MBF, myocardial blood flow; PET, positron emission tomography; TAC, time activity curve.

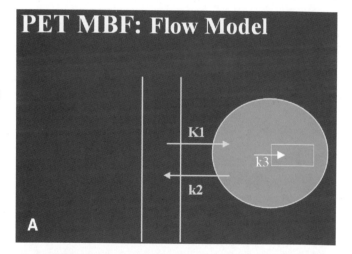

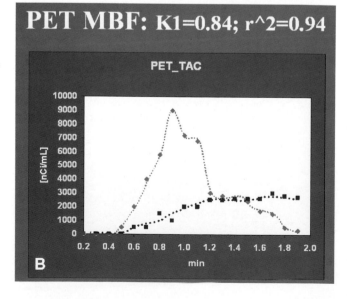

Although well-accepted and extensively validated models exist for N-13 ammonia[10–12] and O-15 water,[3,13–15] the same is not true for rubidium-82, for which models have been published[16,17] but generally have not been widely adopted.

Cyclotron Tracers and Kinetic Models

Radiolabeled O-15 water has been used extensively both for human and animal studies to measure myocardial blood flow.[3,13–15] Image quality, as well as the requirement for an on-site cyclotron, have been problems for the tracer, which has a very short half-life (~120 seconds). Recently a single compartment exponential decay model for flow was combined with factor and cluster analysis to help improve image quality while at the same time accurately obtaining quantitative measurements of myocardial blood flow.[18] Validation studies appear promising and there is even a study using a porcine model in which not only transmural but endocardial and epicardial blood flow measurements were obtained.[18] Water is a freely diffusible molecule, so correction for extraction fraction per se is not required, though a correction factor for tissue water exchangeable volume has been incorporated into at least one commonly employed model.[18] Whether or not this parameter is useful for determination of myocardial scar is a controversial issue[19,20] and remains to be determined. The principal advantage of O-15 water is its brief half-life, which enables multiple measurements of MBF to be made in a short period of time—a feature that has primarily research but also clinical relevance.

N-13 ammonia also requires an on-site cyclotron for production and use since its half-life is ~10 minutes. The relatively short half-life permits multiple flow determination to be made in a relatively short period, but not nearly as rapidly as that with O-15 water. Typically 3–5 half-times must elapse before another measurement can be made, so even with a 10-minute half-life, at least 30 and preferably 50 minutes are required between successive flow measurements. Since ammonia is trapped in the myocardium by the glutamine synthase reaction, image quality is excellent and measurements of myocardial blood flow, especially at low flows, are very good and generally superior to that of O-15 water. Formal head-to-head comparisons of N-13 ammonia and O-15 water have yielded comparable values of absolute MBF in the same individual under a variety of flow conditions.[21,22] The single exception to this statement is at low flow where N-13 ammonia appears to have an advantage over O-15 water when radiolabeled microspheres are used as the gold standard.[21,22]

A two-compartment tracer kinetic model is commonly employed for absolute measurements of MBF with N-13 ammonia, with K1 being the parameter that reflects flow.[10,11] It should be noted that at high flow N-13 ammonia, like other extractable tracers, is not taken up in the myocardium in direct proportion to blood flow, so it is necessary to correct values of K1 for roll-off at high flow rates.[12] The tracer kinetic model has been implemented on a pixel-by-pixel basis in order to provide parametric K1 images (Figures 4.5A and B), which, in contrast to delayed summed images of tracer activity, provide a direct picture of MBF.[11] As noted, however, values of K1 require correction at high flows in order to compensate for incomplete tracer extraction. The results obtained compare quite favorably to those obtained with radiolabeled microspheres over a wide range of flows.[11] Thus, were it not for the requirement of an on-site cyclotron, this tracer would be the agent of choice among presently available ones for quantitative imaging of myocardial blood flow.

It also is worth noting that the trapping of N-13 ammonia has been reported as an indicator of myocardial cell viability because of its dependence on the glutamine synthase reaction.[23] This same phenomenon, however, may also account for the fact that parametric images of MBF may differ from static summed images obtained late in the data acquisition[11] which do not require tracer kinetic modeling to obtain. Accordingly, for N-13 ammonia measurements of MBF, parametric images are preferred to delayed summed images, which at times may be misleading especially with respect to relative differences in regional MBF.[11] Similar differences

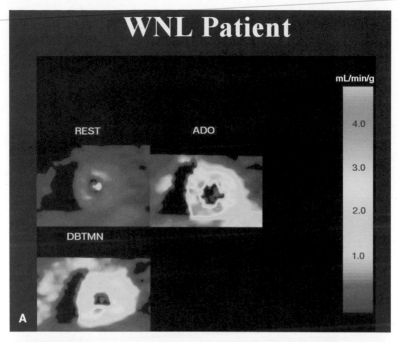

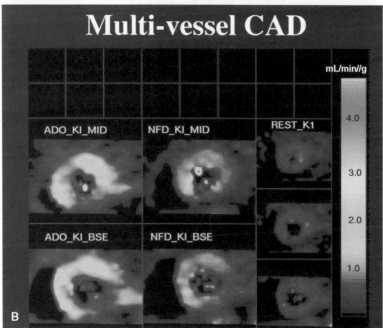

FIGURE 4.5 See color figure on website. (*A*) Shown here is a series of parametric K1 images from a normal subject. The images are of excellent quality and are quantitative in nature. Bright colors correspond to high flows, as expected with Adenosine, and cooler colors correspond to intermediate (*green*) and lower (*blue*) flows as anticipated with dobutamine and at rest, respectively. (*B*) Shown here is a series of parametric K1 images from a patient with multi-vessel CAD. The images are of excellent quality and are quantitative in nature. Although the greatest relative reduction in flow is in the posterolateral region in both Adenosine and nifedipine condition, the remaining myocardial segments also exhibit blunted flow responses to these coronary vasodilators; findings are consistent with angiographic evidence in this patient of triple-vessel CAD. ADO, Adenosine; CAD, coronary artery disease; DBTMN, dobutamine; NFD, nifedipine; WNL, within normal limits.

between early and late tracer distribution have been reported for rubidium-82, and in the past have been employed to distinguish ischemic but viable myocardium from scar[24] (see below).

Rubidium Generator

Rubidium-82 is a decay product of strontium-82 and has a half-life of ~75 seconds. Commercial systems are available that permit the strontium generator to be eluted in a closed system and a calibrated dose injected into the patient without actual technologist handling of the syringe. The advantage of such systems is that they can be shipped to PET imaging centers that do not have cyclotron facilities and generally last ~1 month before the parent nuclide decays away. Tracer quality, however, has been reported to decline as the expiration date draws near, so image quality with a fresh generator often is superior to that with an older one. The images also generally are not as good as those obtained with N-13 ammonia, but for installations without a cyclotron the advantages are generally felt to outweigh the loss in image quality.

Quantitative tracer kinetic models for rubidium have also been published,[17,25] but have not gained wide use either in the clinical or in experimental settings. This likely reflects the fact that research centers have cyclotrons and so prefer O-15 water or N-13 ammonia, which are superior tracers of MBF. In clinical operations the images generally are read qualitatively, so tracer kinetic models are not employed. Since the initial myocardial extraction and retention of the tracer, which is not linear at high flow, depends on the sodium-potassium pump, it has been found that regions of myocardium with substantial fraction of scar tend to lose the tracer faster than viable regions.[24] Accordingly, after waiting for blood pool clearance of the agent (~80 seconds following tracer injection), regions of myocardium with scar show reduced tracer uptake with defects on early images (obtained from ~1.5–3.5 minute post injection), which appear to worsen with time or appear de novo on delayed images (obtained from ~4–8 minutes post tracer injection). In contrast, ischemic but viable myocardium may also show reduced tracer uptake. However, since the sodium-potassium pumps are functioning in such regions, tracer washout is similar to that of normal myocardium and hence defects remain stable with time. Obviously, if only one set of images is obtained at an intermediate time point, such information may be lost or, worse still, the image may reflect the sum of both processes and hence has the potential to either minimize or exaggerate the extent of flow deficit, if any. Finally, the diagnostic accuracy of the approach to determine myocardial viability using sequential myocardial images of Rb82 has recently been challenged.[26]

New Tracers

As noted above, image quality with rubidium-82 may be problematic, and high quality images with N-13 ammonia require cyclotron facilities. Accordingly, there is a need for a myocardial flow tracer that not only produces high quality images but also could be combined with an appropriate tracer kinetic model to obtain quantitative measurements of myocardial blood flow. Since there are ample facilities to delivery F-18–labeled FDG, an F-18–labeled tracer of MBF would be a very desirable imaging agent.

Recently, Shoup et al.[27] have reported the synthesis of F-18-FCPHA (*trans*-9-^{18}F-fluoro-3,4-methyleneheptadecanoic acid), an F-18–labeled fatty acid that may be useful not only to assess myocardial viability by measuring free fatty acid (FFA) metabolism, but also appears to be useful as a tracer of MBF during its initial distribution in the myocardium. Thus, these authors have proposed that with a single tracer injection, high quality quantitative measurements of both MBF and FFA metabolism could be made, which would allow for improved assessment of myocardial viability and metabolism. Further, since F-18-FCPHA is trapped in the myocardium and not metabolized, gated images could easily be obtained following dynamic tracer acquisition and thereby provide accurate measurements of left ventricular volumes, stroke work, and ejection fraction, which would provide an even more complete characterization of the functional status of the heart. Additional experimental work will be required to determine if the theoretical advantages of this compound can be realized in clinical practice. Finally, a report of rat experiments of another promising F-18 labeled MBF tracer also has appeared recently.[27a]

Another tracer that is not new and that requires a cyclotron for production, namely, C-11-acetate, has been employed both for determination of myocardial oxygen consumption (MVO_2) and in conjunction with various tracer kinetic models for MBF.[28–33] Although the use of this tracer for measurement of MBF remains largely experimental and generally is not employed to measure MBF, despite reports of the potential to do so, it has gained wide acceptance as a useful tracer of MVO_2. After intravenous injection and a brief initial delay (~3–5 minutes) to permit initial accumulation and early rapid washout of the tracer from the myocardium, a period of monoexponential decline in myocardial tracer activity follows. The slope of this line, which is linear when fit to a simple natural log function, is termed Kmono and has been shown to provide a good estimate of flux through the Krebs tricarboxylic acid (TCA) cycle and hence MVO_2.[29,32,34] The ability to measure MVO_2 noninvasively and in quantitative terms is extremely helpful when combined with measurements of MBF and left ventricular (LV) contractile function in performing physiological studies of the coronary circulation in human subjects as well as in animal models. Measurement of MVO_2 with C-11 acetate has also been proposed as a method for assessment of myocardial viability, which some have reported is superior to that of F-18-FDG.[35–37] Thus, C-11 acetate is a valuable PET tracer that permits quantitative estimation of MVO_2 and may also be useful for assessment of both MBF and myocardial viability.

Clinical Indications

The sensitivity and specificity of PET myocardial perfusion imaging for detection of coronary artery disease has been looked at by a number of authors. Results of nine studies involving 855 patients have be summarized by Gould[38] and show sensitivity and specificity of 95%. Our own experience in a smaller series of patients (N = 20, 55 coronary vessels analyzed), in which quantitative coronary arteriography was employed as the "gold standard" and compared with quantitative measurements of myocardial blood flow at rest and with Adenosine stress, demonstrated high negative predictive accuracy (91%) and very good positive (75%) and overall (78%) predictive accuracy for detection of hemodynamically significant coronary artery stenoses.[11]

The results of larger series summarized by Gould were obtained, for the most part, based on qualitative interpretation of the images. Quantitative interpretation requires appropriate software, which unfortunately is not routinely available but can be obtained from a European supplier, and development of a normal database for both rest and pharmacologically stimulated (Adenosine or dipyridamole) MBF. Since rest MBF varies widely even among normal subjects and depends on a variety of factors, including, but not limited to, classical determinants of myocardial oxygen demand (i.e., heart rate, preload, afterload, and contractility), it may at times be difficult to define what is normal resting MBF. Further, the traditional flow reserve ratio (MBFstim/MBFrest) is quite sensitive to its denominator, so it may not provide a physiologically meaningful measure of how much MBF can increase in response to an increase in myocardial oxygen demand. Since the heart lives on oxygen supplied by MBF, there is an important difference between a flow reserve ratio of 3X based on an increase in rest MBF from 0.5 mL/min/g to 1.5 mL/min/g with stress, and the same ratio based on an increase in rest flow from 1.0 mL/min/g to 3.0 mL/min/g with stress. The former case may correspond to myocardial hibernation with limited capacity to augment MBF in response to stress, and the latter reflects a normal physiological state. Nonetheless, both have the same flow reserve ratio, which is why we have found it preferable to consider flow reserve in terms of maximal, absolute MBF achieved with Adenosine stimulation rather than the ratio MBFstim/MBFrest.[11]

At the present time, clinically accepted indications for myocardial perfusion imaging (MPI) with PET include the following: (1) obese patients in whom standard SPECT MPI is likely to result in an ambiguous or nondiagnostic study as a result of soft tissue attenuation; (2) to help further evaluate a patient in whom a SPECT MPI study has already been done with ambiguous results; (3) to precisely define absolute myocardial flow reserve in a specific vascular territory in a patient with known coronary artery disease, especially in the setting of multi-vessel disease (typically with prior coronary artery bypass graft [CABG] or percutaneous coronary intervention [PCI]) or prior myocardial infarction—this indication requires the ability to make quantitative measurements of MBF; and (4) a rest MBF measurement to be used in conjunction with PET FDG tracer uptake to assess myocardial viability.

The role of PET MPI *vis-à-vis* other related imaging modalities should also be considered in the context of the above-mentioned clinical indications. Major competing modalities include multislice CT scanning (MSCT) and magnetic resonance imaging (MRI). In terms of routine, clinically available studies, both MSCT and MRI provide superior anatomical information about the heart in comparison with PET, which is primarily a physiological, and therefore fundamentally different, modality. Nonetheless, both MSCT and MRI are capable of routinely producing multi-gated images of the left and right ventricles, and thus qualitative and quantitative assessment of contractile function of each. Multi-gated PET images either of N-13 ammonia or FDG are also capable of providing comparable information concerning left ventricular function.

However, for assessment of coronary artery disease, MSCT has a number of limitations at present, which include: (1) requirement for regular cardiac rhythm; (2) requirement for beta blocker administration to slow the heart to 70's to 80's if greater than that which some patients may not be able to tolerate; (3) radiation and contrast doses similar to that of invasive coronary ateriography; and (4) not infrequent inability to estimate stenosis severity caused by limits of spatial resolution or presence of calcium or stent in the vessel at the stenosis site. The inability to determine the physiological significance of a coronary stenosis then often results in a referral for an imaging stress test (PET, SPECT, or echo) to answer the question. It is also fair to note that at times the traffic moves in the opposite direction, namely, from ambiguous SPECT or echo stress result to an attempt to clarify the situation by MSCT. In that sense the modalities may be complementary, even though they provide fundamentally different information. MRI coronary arteriography[39] and myocardial perfusion studies also have been reported but remain experimental or very limited in availability at the present time. This is not true of MRI for determination of myocardial viability,[40] which is gaining in both availability and popularity at present, and because of its superior spatial resolution and absence of radiation and iodinated contrast requirement, may eclipse other currently available imaging modalities for this indication. It is worth noting that gadolinium, which is used as a contrast agent in MRI viability studies, has been reported to cause renal failure[41] and so presents a risk to patients with coexistent chronic renal disease.

Research applications have been numerous and include studies of coronary endothelial and microvascular function in a variety of experimental settings. Physiological studies of coronary collateral function, coronary "steal," and MBF determinants of contractile responses to inotropic agents such as dobutamine all have been reported, to name but a few.[42–46]

Summary

PET MPI is becoming an increasingly useful modality for clinical assessment of MBF and flow reserve. More widespread dissemination of the technology has resulted from PET imaging advances in clinical oncology. This has fueled the demand for clinical PET scanners and the commercial development of generator delivery systems for rubidium-82, which obviate the need for an on-site cyclotron. The same is true of FDG, which plays an important role in clinical oncology but also is widely used to assess myocardial viability. PET MPI still has yet to reach its full potential since rubidium images are not always optimal, and there is still no widely available and accepted model and software for true quantitative analysis of absolute MBF with the tracer. Nonetheless, improved F-18–based tracers may be available in the not too distant future. Moreover, newer PET/CT scanners may make it possible to combine in one exam the anatomical information obtained with MSCT with the relevant functional information on MBF obtained with PET MPI, and thereby provide a complete anatomical/physiological evaluation of the patient's coronary circulation with a single study.

REFERENCES

1. Gould KL, Schelbert HR, Phelps ME, Hoffman EJ. Noninvasive assessment of coronary stenoses with myocardial perfusion imaging during pharmacologic coronary vasodilatation. V. Detection of 47 percent diameter coronary stenosis with intravenous nitrogen-13 ammonia and emission-computed tomography in intact dogs. *Am J Cardiol.* 1979; 43:200–208.
2. Schelbert HR, Phelps ME, Huang SC, et al. N-13 ammonia as an indicator of myocardial blood flow. *Circulation.* 1981; 63:1259–1272.
3. Bergmann SR, Fox KA, Rand AL, et al. Quantification of regional myocardial blood flow in vivo with H215O. *Circulation.* 1984; 70:724–733.
4. Goldstein RA, Mullani NA, Marani SK, Fisher DJ, Gould KL, O'Brien HA Jr. Myocardial perfusion with rubidium-82. II. Effects of metabolic and pharmacologic interventions. *J Nucl Med.* 1983; 24:907–915.
5. Mullani NA, Goldstein RA, Gould KL, et al. Myocardial perfusion with rubidium-82. I. Measurement of extraction fraction and flow with external detectors. *J Nucl Med.* 1983; 24:898–906.
6. Cook GJ, Fogelman I. The role of positron emission tomography in the management of bone metastases. *Cancer.* 2000; 88:2927–2933.
7. Isasi CR, Lu P, Blaufox MD. A metaanalysis of 18F-2-deoxy-2-fluoro-D-glucose positron emission tomography in the staging and restaging of patients with lymphoma. *Cancer.* 2005; 104:1066–1074.
8. Wiering B, Krabbe PF, Jager GJ, Oyen WJ, Ruers TJ. The impact of fluor-18-deoxyglucose-positron emission tomography in the management of colorectal liver metastases. *Cancer.* 2005; 104:2658–2670.
9. Yano Y, Cahoon JL, Budinger TF. A precision flow-controlled Rb-82 generator for bolus or constant-infusion studies of the heart and brain. *J Nucl Med.* 1981; 22:1006–1010.
10. Hutchins GD, Schwaiger M, Rosenspire KC, Krivokapich J, Schelbert H, Kuhl DE. Noninvasive quantification of regional blood flow in the human heart using N-13 ammonia and dynamic positron emission tomographic imaging. *J Am Coll Cardiol.* 1990; 15:1032–1042.
11. Gewirtz H, Skopicki HA, Abraham SA, et al. Quantitative PET measurements of regional myocardial blood flow: Observations in humans with ischemic heart disease. *Cardiology.* 1997; 88:62–70.
12. Gewirtz H, Fischman AJ, Abraham SA, Gilson M, Strauss HW, Alpert NM. Positron emission tomographic measurements of absolute regional myocardial blood flow permits identification of nonviable myocardium in patients with chronic myocardial infarction. *J Am Coll Cardiol.* 1994; 23:851–859.
13. Bol A, Melin J, Vanoverschelde J, Weinheimer CJ, Walsh MN. Direct comparison of 13-N-ammonia and 15-O-water estimates of perfusion and quantification of regional myocardial blood flow by microspheres. *Circulation.* 1993; 87:512–525.
14. Bergmann SR, Herrero P, Markham J, Weinheimer CJ, Walsh MN. Noninvasive quantitation of myocardial blood flow in human subjects with oxygen-15-labeled water and positron emission tomography. *J Am Coll Cardiol.* 1989; 14:639–652.
15. Merlet P, Mazoyer B, Hittinger L, et al. Assessment of coronary reserve in man: Comparison between positron emission tomography with oxygen-15-labeled water and intracoronary Doppler technique. *J Nucl Med.* 1993; 34:1899–1904.
16. Herrero P, Markham J, Shelton ME, Weinheimer CJ, Bergmann SR. Noninvasive quantification of regional myocardial perfusion with rubidium-82 and positron emission tomography. Exploration of a mathematical model. *Circulation.* 1990; 82:1377–1386.
17. El Fakhri G, Sitek A, Guerin B, Kijewski MF, Di Carli MF, Moore SC. Quantitative dynamic cardiac 82Rb PET using generalized factor and compartment analyses. *J Nucl Med.* 2005; 46:1264–1271.
18. Rimoldi O, Schafers KP, Boellaard R, et al. Quantification of subendocardial and subepicardial blood flow using 15O-labeled water and PET: Experimental validation. *J Nucl Med.* 2006; 47:163–172.
19. Herrero P, Staudenherz A, Walsh JF, Gropler RJ, Bergmann SR. Heterogeneity of myocardial perfusion provides the physiological basis of perfusable tissue index. *J Nucl Med.* 1995; 36:320–327.
20. Gerber BL, Melin JA, Bol A, et al. Nitrogen-13-ammonia and oxygen-15-water estimates of absolute myocardial perfusion in left ventricular ischemic dysfunction. *J Nucl Med.* 1998; 39:1655–1662.
21. Bol A, Melin JA, Vanoverschelde JL, et al. Direct comparison of [13N]ammonia and [15O]water estimates of perfusion with quantification of regional myocardial blood flow by microspheres. *Circulation.* 1993; 87:512–525.
22. Chareonthaitawee P, Christenson SD, Anderson JL, et al. Reproducibility of measurements of regional myocardial blood flow in a model of coronary artery disease: Comparison of H215O and 13NH3 PET techniques. *J Nucl Med.* 2006; 47:1193–1201.
23. Kitsiou AN, Bacharach SL, Bartlett ML, et al. 13N-ammonia myocardial blood flow and uptake: Relation to functional outcome of asynergic regions after revascularization. *J Am Coll Cardiol.* 1999; 33:678–686.
24. Gould K. Assessing myocardial viability. In: *Coronary Artery Stenosis and Reversing Atherosclerosis.* 2nd ed. New York: Arnold/Oxford University Press; 1999:340–349.
25. Herrero P, Markham J, Shelton ME, Bergmann SR. Implementation and evaluation of a two-compartment model for quantification of myocardial perfusion with rubidium-82 and positron emission tomography. *Circ Res.* 1992; 70:496–507.

26. Stankewicz MA, Mansour CS, Eisner RL, et al. Myocardial viability assessment by PET: (82)Rb defect washout does not predict the results of metabolic-perfusion mismatch. *J Nucl Med.* 2005; 46:1602–1609.

27. Shoup TM, Elmaleh DR, Bonab AA, Fischman AJ. Evaluation of trans-9-18F-fluoro-3,4-methyleneheptade-canoic acid as a PET tracer for myocardial fatty acid imaging. *J Nucl Med.* 2005; 46:297–304.

27a. Huisman MC, Higuchi T, Reder S, et al. Initial Characterization of an 18F-Labeled Myocardial Perfusion Tracer. *J Nucl Med.* 2008; 49:630–636.

28. Porenta G, Cherry S, Czernin J, et al. Noninvasive determination of myocardial blood flow, oxygen consumption and efficiency in normal humans by carbon-11 acetate positron emission tomography imaging. *Eur J Nucl Med.* 1999; 26:1465–1474.

29. Klein LJ, Visser FC, Knaapen P, et al. Carbon-11 acetate as a tracer of myocardial oxygen consumption. *Eur J Nucl Med.* 2001; 28:651–668.

30. Sun KT, Yeatman LA, Buxton DB, et al. Simultaneous measurement of myocardial oxygen consumption and blood flow using [1-carbon-11]acetate. *J Nucl Med.* 1998; 39:272–280.

31. Sun KT, Chen K, Huang SC, et al. Compartment model for measuring myocardial oxygen consumption using [1-11C]acetate. *J Nucl Med.* 1997; 38:459–466.

32. Armbrecht JJ, Buxton DB, Schelbert HR. Validation of [1-11C]acetate as a tracer for noninvasive assessment of oxidative metabolism with positron emission tomography in normal, ischemic, postischemic, and hyperemic canine myocardium. *Circulation.* 1990; 81:1594–1605.

33. Sciacca RR, Akinboboye O, Chou RL, Epstein S, Bergmann SR. Measurement of myocardial blood flow with PET using 1-11C-acetate. *J Nucl Med.* 2001; 42:63–70.

34. Armbrecht JJ, Buxton DB, Brunken RC, Phelps ME, Schelbert HR. Regional myocardial oxygen consumption determined noninvasively in humans with [1-11C]acetate and dynamic positron tomography. *Circulation.* 1989; 80:863–872.

35. Rubin PJ, Lee DS, Davila-Roman VG, et al. Superiority of C-11 acetate compared with F-18 fluorodeoxyglucose in predicting myocardial functional recovery by positron emission tomography in patients with acute myocardial infarction. *Am J Cardiol.* 1996; 78:1230–1235.

36. Gropler RJ, Geltman EM, Sampathkumaran K, et al. Comparison of carbon-11-acetate with fluorine-18-fluorodeoxyglucose for delineating viable myocardium by positron emission tomography. *J Am Coll Cardiol.* 1993; 22:1587–1597.

37. Gropler RJ, Siegel BA, Sampathkumaran K, et al. Dependence of recovery of contractile function on maintenance of oxidative metabolism after myocardial infarction. *J Am Coll Cardiol.* 1992; 19:989–997.

38. Gould K. PET perfusion imaging. In: *Coronary Artery Stenosis and Reversing Atherosclerosis.* 2nd ed. New York: Arnold/Oxford Univeristy Press; 1999: 221–223.

39. Kim WY, Danias PG, Stuber M, et al. Coronary magnetic resonance angiography for the detection of coronary stenoses. *N Engl J Med.* 2001; 345:1863–1869.

40. Kim RJ, Lima JA, Chen EL, et al. Fast 23Na magnetic resonance imaging of acute reperfused myocardial infarction. Potential to assess myocardial viability. *Circulation.* 1997; 95:1877–1885.

41. Ergun I, Keven K, Uruc I, et al. The safety of gadolinium in patients with stage 3 and 4 renal failure. *Nephrol Dial Transplant.* 2006; 21:697–700.

42. Skopicki HA, Abraham SA, Picard MH, et al. Effects of dobutamine at maximally tolerated dose on myocardial blood flow in humans with ischemic heart disease [published erratum appears in Circulation 97(4):414]. *Circulation.* 1997; 96:3346–3352.

43. Skopicki HA, Abraham SA, Weissman NJ, et al. Factors influencing regional myocardial contractile response to inotropic stimulation. Analysis in humans with stable ischemic heart disease. *Circulation.* 1996; 94:643–650.

44. Huggins GS, Pasternak RC, Alpert NM, et al. Effects of short-term treatment of hyperlipidemia on coronary vasodilator function and myocardial perfusion in regions having substantial impairment of baseline dilator reverse [see comments]. *Circulation.* 1998; 98:1291–1296.

45. Holmvang G, Fry S, Skopicki HA, et al. Relation between coronary "steal" and contractile function at rest in collateral-dependent myocardium of humans with ischemic heart disease. *Circulation.* 1999; 99:2510–2516.

46. Huisman MC, Higuchi T, Reder S, et al. Initial characterization of an 18F-labeled myocardial perfusion tracer. *J Nucl Med.* 2008; 49:630–636.

4.4 PET Viability Studies

Henry Gewirtz

Definitions of Myocardial Hibernation, Stunning, and Viability

As in any area of medicine, especially one that has more than its share of controversy, it is important to define terms if one is to have any hope of making sense of the problem. Although the pathophysiology of myocardial hibernation and stunning remains controversial, the following points are clear. Both entities share in common impaired contractile function of the left ventricle. Classically, stunning was thought to differ from hibernation since the former was characterized by relatively normal myocardial blood flow and myocardial oxygen consumption out of proportion to the decreased contractile function of the myocardium involved.[1–4] In contrast, hibernation classically was thought to involve a matched reduction in myocardial blood flow, contractile function, and oxygen consumption.[1–4] In patients with ischemic heart disease and in animal models,[5,6] PET studies have demonstrated that both patterns of myocardial blood flow and impairment contractile function may exist, sometimes even in the same subject.[7] It also appears to be true that chronic stunning often precedes hibernation.[8,9] It has also been suggested that hibernation may occur in the absence of prior stunning.[1,6,10] Further, the underlying histopathology is also somewhat controversial but has been characterized by glycogen accumulation, myocyte dedifferentiation, increased interstitial fibrosis, and in some but not all series, evidence of myocyte loss by apoptosis.[1,11–15] A detailed review of the data relevant to this controversy is beyond the scope of this chapter. What is important for the purposes of this review is that both states, however arrived at, are characterized by dysfunctional myocardium, and both have the potential to improve with myocardial revascularization. Thus, there is a need to distinguish viable myocardium (i.e., hibernating or stunned) from nonviable myocardium, which is largely composed of scar tissue.

Myocardial viability, in turn, has been defined in one of two ways. The first employs what may be termed a cellular definition. This approach rests on the notion that accumulation of various radiotracers (e.g., Thallium, technetium-99m-sestamibi, rubidium-82) requires cellular concentrating mechanisms such as the sodium-potassium ATPase pump (Thallium, rubidium-82) or the electrochemical gradient of intact mitochondria (Tc-99m-sestamibi), and since these pumps require energy to function, a cell that can accumulate the tracer of interest must be viable.[16,17] An alternate and perhaps more widely accepted definition holds that viable myocardium is best characterized by return or improvement of contractile function following coronary revascularization.[18–20] The argument in support of this definition runs to the effect that what is important to the individual is whether or not myocardium with impaired contractility is functionally improved when it is revascularized. A surrogate end point such as tracer accumulation, although it is a marker for an energy-requiring metabolic process, has a lesser oxygen consumption requirement (only about 20% of basal MVO_2) than that of contraction, which ultimately is what the patient lives or dies by. The argument against this definition is the often subjective nature of contractile function assessment, typically by echocardiography, though gated MRI has also been used, and the fact that myocardial tethering, interstitial fibrosis, and cellular dedifferentiation all may occur, so that even if the segment(s) in question are successfully revascularized, contractile function still may not be restored depending on when contractile function is reevaluated. Nonetheless, the improvement of contractile function of the left ventricle following coronary revascularization remains the most widely accepted definition of myocardial "viability," and those tests that best predict this outcome are thought to be the best for viability assessment.

Methodology

SPECT (TI , MIBI)

The first radionuclide tracer to be employed for the assessment of myocardial viability was Thallium. The tracer has some properties of a potassium analog, so accumulation of the tracer in the myocardium is thought to be indicative of functioning Na-K ATPase pumps. The tracer is typically injected with the patient at rest, and images of the heart are obtained 10–15 minutes later and again at periods varying from 4–24 hours later. The utility of the 24-hour time point, however, is controversial and there are data that show that whatever redistribution (see below) is destined to occur does so within 4 hours and that waiting longer to image does not improve upon this, especially since 24-hour images are count poor and may be very difficult to interpret.[21]

Since the initial distribution of Thallium tends to be blood flow dependent and late images mark the viable Na-K ATPase pump pool, initial defects that appear to resolve on delayed images are most specific for myocardial viability. The original description of this finding was reported in 1979 prior to widespread appreciation of the concepts of myocardial hibernation and stunning, although the report in fact noted that such segments must have both low flow and viability[22] (i.e., exhibit what is now termed myocardial hibernation). Since then it also has been shown that milder fixed defects on Thallium scans also have substantial viable myocardium and are likely to improve contractile function upon successful revascularization.[21]

When improvement of left ventricular contractile function, either global or segmental, is used as the "gold standard" for myocardial viability, the rest redistribution Thallium study, as it is commonly known, has been shown to be quite sensitive for detection of viable myocardium, but specificity and hence overall predictive accuracy has been variable with a range of roughly 60%–75%, though with high negative predictive accuracy in the range of 90%–95%.[23–25] Stated in other terms, if the rest redistribution Thallium study is negative for myocardial viability, then it is highly unlikely such segments will recover or improve function upon revascularization. In contrast, if the segment either shows definite redistribution or a fixed but relatively mild defect and hence viability, it is more likely than not that contraction will improve after revascularization, especially if the segment is hypokinetic as opposed to akinetic or dyskinetic.[24]

Although rest Tc-99m-MIBI scans are less commonly employed for viability assessment, reported results[23] have been comparable to that of Thallium, notwithstanding the fact that MIBI does not exhibit appreciable redistribution. Rest MIBI scans obtained 1 hour post tracer injection have been shown to closely resemble redistribution Thallium images and hence provide comparable information regarding cellular viability.[23] The performance of the tracer in predicting recovery of contractile function of myocardium considered to be viable by this technique likewise is comparable to that of Thallium.[23] The positive and negative predictive accuracies for recovery of contractile function in the series of Udelson et al.[23] was good (Thallium positive predictive accuracy 75% vs. MIBI 80%, and negative predictive accuracy 92% and 96%, respectively). However, as noted above other reports have not been as favorable for Thallium[24,25] with respect to positive predictive accuracy.

A newer approach, which has been employed in both Japan and Europe for assessment of myocardial viability, has been to combine SPECT imaging of the I-123–labeled fatty acid analog beta-methyl-p-[(123)I]-iodophenyl-pentadecanoic acid (BMIPP) with either tetrofosmin or MIBI to evaluate the relationship between myocardial perfusion (MIBI or tetrofosmin) and fatty acid metabolism. The pattern of reduced BMIPP uptake vis-á-vis myocardial perfusion in small series has shown moderate (~70%–75%) predictive accuracy for recovery of contractile function following coronary revascularization.[26,27] Additional large-scale clinical trials will be required to determine the true value of this approach for identification of myocardial viability in regions with contractile dysfunction and their recovery following revascularization.

PET (FDG/NH3, C-11 Acetate-MVO₂, Fatty Acid Tracers)

The established "gold standard" for assessment of myocardial viability has been the PET FDG/myocardial perfusion study (N-13 ammonia or O-15 water). The technique was originally described by Schelbert et al.[28] and is currently employed by many PET laboratories around the world.[7,29–34] Sensitivity and specificity for the method when recovery of contractile function is used as the basis for evaluation is on the order of 85% if optimized criteria for FDG uptake and rest myocardial blood flow are employed.[34] The FDG part of the study requires either an oral glucose load followed approximately 30 minutes later by FDG injection and then image acquisition 45 minutes after that. The euglycemic, hyperinsulinemic technique requires more time and closer patient monitoring, but is felt by many to produce superior images and is widely employed in European laboratories.[32] It is possible with appropriate glucose loading protocols and supplemental insulin treatment to obtain diagnostic images in most diabetic patients.[35]

The pattern of tracer uptake that has been found to best predict recovery of contractile function is the so-called FDG–blood flow "mismatch." Thus, in mismatch segments myocardial blood flow is reduced relative to FDG uptake such that myocardial FDG activity appears increased in a region with a flow defect on the perfusion image (N-13 ammonia or O-15 water). It should be noted that SPECT imaging with Tc-99m-MIBI (or tetrofosmin) may be used for the perfusion assessment in those laboratories with a PET camera but without access to a cyclotron to produce N-13 ammonia or O-15 water. An example of a PET FDG blood flow mismatch is shown in Figure 4.6.

Although the pathophysiologic basis for FDG–blood flow mismatch is not fully defined, it appears to depend at least in part on upregulation of the GLUT-4 glucose tranporter and its translocation to the cell membrane in hibernating or stunned myocardium. Since increased myocyte glycogen content has been described in chronic hibernation,[10,36,37] it is unclear if enhanced glucose uptake by these cells reflects increased storage of glucose as glycogen or increased anaerobic metabolism of glucose. Although increased anaerobic glucose metabolism

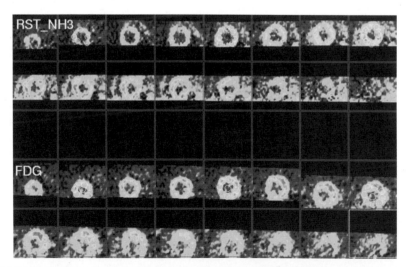

FIGURE 4.6 Shown here are matched short axis images (*apex at upper left corner, base at lower right of each sequence*) of rest myocardial blood flow and FDG uptake in a patient with known ischemic heart disease. Note the classic "mismatch" pattern with greatly reduced flow (*pale green colors at apical and mid LV levels in top row of RST_NH3*) with well-preserved FDG uptake (*yellow-red colors*) in these same segments (*top row of FDG*). FDG, fluorodeoxyglucose; LV, left ventricular; RST_NH3, rest myocardial blood flow.

is a feature of acute myocardial ischemia, it likely does not play a role in the chronic adjustment of the myocardium to reduction in myocardial blood flow.[6,11,38]

Alternative approaches to myocardial viability assessment with PET tracers have included the use of C-11–labeled fatty acids and acetate.[39–42] Although there are reports that indicate C-11 acetate, which is used to measure myocardial oxygen consumption, the *sine qua non* of myocardial viability, may be superior to FDG for viability assessment,[39,40] the method has not gained wide acceptance, at least in part because it is cyclotron dependent and thus limited in its applicability. The same is true of C-11–labeled fatty acids, typically C-11-palmitate.

Echocardiography (Dobutamine Stress)

Dobutamine stress echocardiography (DSE) has been a frequently employed method used to assess myocardial viability. It has the advantages of being widely available, noninvasive, relatively inexpensive, and it directly images the outcome of interest, namely, regional myocardial contraction. Thus, an echocardiogram is obtained at baseline and with low and higher dose dobutamine stress. The so-called biphasic response to dobutamine has been thought to be the most specific and best indicator of recovery of segmental function.[43,44] This response relies upon the presence of some contractile reserve in hibernating or stunned myocardium such that with low dose inotropic stimulation contractile function improves, whereas at a higher dose myocardial flow reserve is inadequate to support the level of increased myocardial oxygen demand. Thus, ischemia ensues and contractile function declines as a result. The fact that the segment is capable of both contractile augmentation and induction of ischemia is taken as double confirmation of myocardial viability. It should be noted that some segments have been shown to improve contraction despite failure to augment with dobutamine stimulation. The reason for this is unclear but may reflect issues related to tethering[45] as well as wall motion assessment in dilated, poorly functioning ventricles with diffuse baseline contractile abnormalities.

A recent study[30] has proposed combining SPECT Thallium imaging with DSE in an effort to overcome the weaknesses of each (i.e., reduced specificity for Thallium and low sensitivity for DSE). In this study of 47 patients, SPECT Thallium alone had high sensitivity for prediction of recovery of LV contractile function post CABG (95%), but low specificity (57%). DSE alone had low sensitivity (63%) but high specificity (89%). When the two methods were sequentially employed (SPECT Thallium then DSE), sensitivity was 89% and specificity improved to 86%. PET FDG in this same patient population had similar sensitivity (89%) and specificity (89%) to the combined approach. The authors concluded that in centers without access to PET imaging that combined SPECT Thallium, DSE was an excellent and comparable alternative for viability assessment.

MRI

MRI has been employed in conjunction with dobutamine stress to assess myocardial viability.[46,47] The approach that was originally employed reflected a technique similar to that employed by echocardiography in that the contractile response to dobutamine was assessed before and after coronary revascularization. A variety of MRI parameters have been employed, such as diastolic and systolic wall thickness at baseline and wall thickening with dobutamine. The diastolic criteria is employed to weed out scar segments that are thinner (<5 mm) than that of normal or viable ones.[46] Other techniques employed include more sophisticated ones, such as tissue tagging and MRI systolic strain analysis, as well as relatively simple ones, such as visual assessment of global and regional contractile function of gated MR images in which appropriate pulse sequences are used to render LV blood bright, thus producing a high resolution, tomographic cineventriculogram.[47]

More recently, these techniques have been combined with or supplanted by gadolinium (Gd) contrast enhanced MR images of the left ventricle.[48–53] It has been demonstrated that gadolinium selectively accumulates in nonviable myocardial regions in delayed contrast-enhanced images of the left ventricle.[48] Further, it has been demonstrated that regions with less delayed enhancement (i.e., more viable myocardium) are more likely to recover contractile function following CABG or after myocardial infarction than those with a greater extent of transmural hyperenhancement.[52,54] The performance of the technique has been compared to dobutamine stress cine MRI and has been shown in at least one study[55] to be very good, though not as good as dobutamine stress cine MRI (sensitivity, specificity, accuracy of 83%,72%,79%, respectively, for contrast enhancement versus 89%, 80%, 86%, respectively, for dobutamine stress cine MRI). Nonetheless, accuracy is excellent for contrast enhancement and the ease of application has made it an increasingly popular technique, though its application to patients with renal insufficiency carries with it the risk of acute renal failure caused by gadolinium.[56]

Clinical Issues

Increased Risk of CABG in Low Ejection Fraction Patients

In the setting of left ventricular failure with markedly reduced ejection fraction (EF) (<30), selection of patients with ischemic heart disease who will benefit from coronary revascularization is problematic. Surgical mortality is increased in such patients, though in a recent series operative mortality was only 3.8% and actuarial survival 94%, 82%, and 68% at 1, 2, and 5 years, respectively, postoperatively in 79 consecutive patients with LVEF $18 \pm 5\%$.[57] Nevertheless, physicians understandably hesitate to recommend surgery for these patients if the prospects for benefit are limited. Accordingly, it is useful to consider the precise indication for surgery (i.e., mortality benefit vs. relief or amelioration of heart failure vs. treatment of medically refractory angina pectoris) since outcomes vary depending on the surgical indication (see below).

Inadequacy of Current Data on Benefits

It has been shown that ischemic heart disease (IHD) patients with low LVEF who are operated on primarily for angina are more likely to obtain symptomatic benefit than those operated on primarily for heart failure.[57,58] Mortality data, however, usually include all patients with IHD and low LVEF and have demonstrated a survival advantage relative to historical controls who are medically treated.[57,58] Further, the study of Mickleborough et al. reported no difference in long-term survival between those operated on primarily for angina versus those for heart failure.[57] Unfortunately, these data are observational and retrospective in nature. There are no data from prospective randomized clinical trials to address this issue. Further, although it has been reported that symptoms of heart failure and angina were improved post CABG in patients with low preoperative LVEF (0.24 ± 0.05), this occurred independent of any improvement in global left ventricular systolic function.[59] There was also no difference in survival in the group that failed to improve LVEF (0.24 ± 0.05 to 0.23 ± 0.06) in comparison with the group that did improve (0.24 ± 0.05 to 0.39 ± 0.10).[59] Accordingly, although patients may feel better and perhaps live longer post CABG in this patient population, the mechanism is not clear and certainly is not dependent upon improvement in LVEF. Prevention of adverse remodeling and possibly increasing electrical stability of the myocardium are potential mechanisms and require investigation, as noted above in a randomized clinical trial in patients with coronary artery disease and severe left ventricular dysfunction. Finally, it is worth noting that the correlation between exercise capacity and LVEF in chronic LV dysfunction is known to be poor,[60,61] so it should not be surprising that improvement in chronic heart failure (CHF) symptoms (or lack thereof) does not correlate well with improvement of LVEF post CABG, which on average is usually only modest (~10 EF units).[62,63]

Summary/Conclusions

Myocardial hibernation and/or chronic stunning are responsible for reversible LV dysfunction in the setting of chronic ischemic heart disease. Retrospective, observational studies indicate that revascularization of such myocardial segments, particularly if they make up a substantial fraction of the left ventricle (30%–50% in some series[62,63]), results in improved survival and symptomatic status compared with medically treated patients with similar impairment of LV contractile function who lack substantial residual viable myocardium. The optimal technique for assessment of myocardial viability in this setting is a work in progress. It depends on a host of factors, not least of which are those that are available in a given center and the expertise of the imaging group(s) involved. The standard recommendation in such situations is to use the imaging technique with which the physicians have the greatest expertise and are most experienced. One must also consider the indication for which CABG/PCI is being contemplated. If heart failure is the issue, then a study that directly measures the recruitable inotropic reserve such as DSE or cine MRI may be preferable to one that focuses more on cellular metabolism. If refractory angina is the clinical problem, then a test of cellular metabolism (e.g., PET FDG with myocardial perfusion imaging) may be best. The role of imaging late hyper-enhancement with gadolinium contrast and MRI is gaining in popularity and may prove to be the most versatile of currently available techniques, though it is by no means perfect. Additional prospective, randomized clinical trials are required both to test the hypothesis that coronary revascularization truly is advantageous in this patient population, and that gadolinium contrast MRI is the optimal way to select such patients for CABG.

REFERENCES

1. Heusch G, Schulz R, Rahimtoola SH. Myocardial hibernation: A delicate balance. *Am J Physiol Heart Circ Physiol*. 2005; 288:H984–H999.
2. Elladi PP, Rahimtoola SH. Myocardial viability and hibernation: Still an incomplete picture. *Ital Heart J*. 2002; 3:279–281.
3. Rahimtoola SH. Chronic myocardial hibernation. *Circulation*. 1994; 89:1907–1908
4. Kloner RA, Bolli R, Marban E, Reinlib L, Braunwald E. Medical and cellular implications of stunning, hibernation, and preconditioning: An NHLBI workshop. *Circulation*. 1998; 97:1848–1867.
5. Canty JMJ, Klocke FJ. Reductions in regional myocardial function at rest in conscious dogs with chronically reduced regional coronary artery pressure. *Circ Res (Suppl II)*. 1987; 61:II-107–II-116.
6. Mills I, Fallon JT, Wrenn D, et al. Adaptive responses of the coronary circulation and myocardium to chronic reduction in perfusion pressure and flow. *Am J Physiol (Heart Circ Physiol 35)*. 1994; 266:H447–H457.
7. Tawakol A, Skopicki HA, Abraham SA, et al. Evidence of reduced resting blood flow in viable myocardial regions with chronic asynergy. *J Am Coll Cardiol*. 2000; 36:2146–2153.
8. Fallavollita J, Canty JJ. Differential 18-F-2-deoxyglucose uptake in viable dysfunctional myocardium with normal resting perfusion: Evidence for chronic stunning in pigs. *Circulation*. 1999; 99:2798–2805.
9. Fallavollita J, Perry B, Canty JJ. 18-F-2-deoxyglucose deposition and regional flow in pigs with chronically dysfunctional myocardium: Evidence for transmural variations in chronic hibernating myocardium. *Circulation*. 1997; 95:1900–1909.
10. Heusch G, Schulz R. Hibernating myocardium: A review. *J Mol Cell Cardiol*. 1996; 28:2359–2372.
11. Ausma J, Thone F, Dispersyn GD, et al. Dedifferentiated cardiomyocytes from chronic hibernating myocardium are ischemia-tolerant. *Mol Cell Biochem*. 1998; 186:159–168.
12. Depre C, Taegtmeyer H. Metabolic aspects of programmed cell survival and cell death in the heart. *Cardiovasc Res*. 2000; 45:538–548.
13. Ausma J, Furst D, Thone F, et al. Molecular changes of titin in left ventricular dysfunction as a result of chronic hibernation. *J Mol Cell Cardiol*. 1995; 27:1203–1212.
14. Ausma J, Cleutjens J, Thone F, Flameng W, Ramaekers F, Borgers M. Chronic hibernating myocardium: Interstitial changes. *Mol Cell Biochem*. 1995; 147:35–42.
15. Schwarz ER, Schaper J, vom Dahl J, et al. Myocyte degeneration and cell death in hibernating human myocardium. *J Am Coll Cardiol*. 1996; 27:1577–1585.
16. Dilsizian V. Myocardial viability: Contractile reserve or cell membrane integrity? [editorial comment]. *J Am Coll Cardiol*. 1996; 28:443–446.
17. Dilsizian V, Bonow RO. Current diagnostic techniques of assessing myocardial viability in patients with hibernating and stunned myocardium [published erratum appears in Circulation 1993 Jun; 87(6):2070]. *Circulation*. 1993; 87:1–20.
18. Vanoverschelde JL, Depre C, Gerber BL, et al. Time course of functional recovery after coronary artery bypass graft surgery in patients with chronic left ventricular ischemic dysfunction. *Am J Cardiol*. 2000; 85:1432–1439.

19. Haas F, Jennen L, Heinzmann U, et al. Ischemically compromised myocardium displays different time-courses of functional recovery: Correlation with morphological alterations? *Eur J Cardiothorac Surg.* 2001; 20:290–298.
20. Mazur W, Nagueh SF. Myocardial viability: Recent developments in detection and clinical significance. *Curr Opin Cardiol.* 2001; 16:277–281.
21. Ragosta M, Beller GA, Watson DD, Kaul S, Gimple LW. Quantitative planar rest-redistribution 201Tl imaging in detection of myocardial viability and prediction of improvement in left ventricular function after coronary bypass surgery in patients with severely depressed left ventricular function. *Circulation.* 1993; 87:1630–1641.
22. Gewirtz H, Beller GA, Strauss HW, et al. Transient defects of resting Thallium scans in patients with coronary artery disease. *Circulation.* 1979; 59:707–713.
23. Udelson JE, Coleman PS, Metherall J, et al. Predicting recovery of severe regional ventricular dysfunction. Comparison of resting scintigraphy with 201Tl and 99mTc-sestamibi. *Circulation.* 1994; 89:2552–2561.
24. Perrone-Filardi P, Pace L, Prastaro M, et al. Assessment of myocardial viability in patients with chronic coronary artery disease. Rest-4-hour-24-hour 201Tl tomography versus dobutamine echocardiography. *Circulation.* 1996; 94:2712–2719.
25. Duncan BH, Ahlberg AW, Levine MG, et al. Comparison of electrocardiographic-gated technetium-99m sestamibi single-photon emission computed tomographic imaging and rest-redistribution Thallium-201 in the prediction of myocardial viability. *Am J Cardiol.* 2000; 85:680–684.
26. Seki H, Toyama T, Higuchi K, et al. Prediction of functional improvement of ischemic myocardium with (123I-BMIPP SPECT and 99mTc-tetrofosmin SPECT imaging: A study of patients with large acute myocardial infarction and receiving revascularization therapy. *Circ J.* 2005; 69:311–319.
27. Hambye AS, Vervaet A, Dobbeleir A. Quantification of 99Tcm-sestamibi and 123I-BMIPP uptake for predicting functional outcome in chronically ischaemic dysfunctional myocardium. *Nucl Med Commun.* 1999; 20:737–745.
28. Tillisch J, Brunken R, Marshall R, et al. Reversibility of cardiac wall-motion abnormalities predicted by positron tomography. *N Engl J Med.* 1986; 314:884–888.
29. Dilsizian V, Perrone-Filardi P, Arrighi JA, et al. Concordance and discordance between stress-redistribution-reinjection and rest-redistribution Thallium imaging for assessing viable myocardium. Comparison with metabolic activity by positron emission tomography. *Circulation.* 1993; 88:941–952.
30. Bax JJ, Maddahi J, Poldermans D, et al. Preoperative comparison of different noninvasive strategies for predicting improvement in left ventricular function after coronary artery bypass grafting. *Am J Cardiol.* 2003; 92:1–4.
31. Lund GK, Freyhoff J, Schwaiger M, et al. Prediction of left ventricular functional recovery by dobutamine echocardiography, F-18 deoxyglucose or 99mTc sestamibi nuclear imaging in patients with chronic myocardial infarction. *Cardiology.* 2002; 98:202–209.
32. Gerber BL, Ordoubadi FF, Wijns W, et al. Positron emission tomography using(18)F-fluoro-deoxyglucose and euglycaemic hyperinsulinaemic glucose clamp: Optimal criteria for the prediction of recovery of post-ischaemic left ventricular dysfunction. Results from the European Community Concerted Action Multicenter study on use of(18)F-fluoro-deoxyglucose Positron Emission Tomography for the Detection of Myocardial Viability. *Eur Heart J.* 2001; 22:1691–1701.
33. McFalls EO, Baldwin D, Kuskowski M, Liow J, Chesler E, Ward HB. Utility of positron emission tomography in predicting improved left ventricular ejection fraction after coronary artery bypass grafting among patients with ischemic cardiomyopathy. *Cardiology.* 2000; 93:105–112.
34. Knuuti MJ, Saraste M, Nuutila P, et al. Myocardial viability: Fluorine-18-deoxyglucose positron emission tomography in prediction of wall motion recovery after revascularization. *Am Heart J.* 1994; 127:785–796.
35. Schoder H, Campisi R, Ohtake T, et al. Blood flow-metabolism imaging with positron emission tomography in patients with diabetes mellitus for the assessment of reversible left ventricular contractile dysfunction. *J Am Coll Cardiol.* 1999; 33:1328–1337.
36. Depre C, Vanoverschelde J, Melin J, et al. Structural and metabolic correlates of the reversibility of chronic left ventricular ischemic dysfunction in humans. *Am J Physiol (Heart Circ Physiol 37).* 1995; 268:H1265–H1275.
37. Gunning MG, Kaprielian RR, Pepper J, et al. The histology of viable and hibernating myocardium in relation to imaging characteristics. *J Am Coll Cardiol.* 2002; 39:428–435.
38. Fedele FA, Gewirtz H, Capone RJ, Sharaf B, Most AS. Metabolic response to prolonged reduction of myocardial blood flow distal to a severe coronary artery stenosis. *Circulation.* 1988; 78:729–735.
39. Rubin PJ, Lee DS, Davila-Roman VG, et al. Superiority of C-11 acetate compared with F-18 fluorodeoxyglucose in predicting myocardial functional recovery by positron emission tomography in patients with acute myocardial infarction. *Am J Cardiol.* 1996; 78:1230–1235.
40. Gropler RJ, Geltman EM, Sampathkumaran K, et al. Comparison of carbon-11-acetate with fluorine-18-fluorodeoxyglucose for delineating viable myocardium by positron emission tomography. *J Am Coll Cardiol.* 1993; 22:1587–1597.
41. Gropler RJ, Siegel BA, Sampathkumaran K, et al. Dependence of recovery of contractile function on maintenance of oxidative metabolism after myocardial infarction. *J Am Coll Cardiol.* 1992; 19:989–997.

42. Bergmann SR, Weinheimer CJ, Markham J, Herrero P. Quantitation of myocardial fatty acid metabolism using PET. *J Nucl Med.* 1996; 37:1723–1730.

43. Cigarroa CG, deFilippi CR, Brickner ME, Alvarez LG, Wait MA, Grayburn PA. Dobutamine stress echocardiography identifies hibernating myocardium and predicts recovery of left ventricular function after coronary revascularization. *Circulation.* 1993; 88:430–436.

44. Marwick T, D'Hondt AM, Baudhuin T, et al. Optimal use of dobutamine stress for the detection and evaluation of coronary artery disease: Combination with echocardiography or scintigraphy, or both? *J Am Coll Cardiol.* 1993; 22:159–167.

45. Chia KK, Picard MH, Skopicki HA, Hung J. Viability of hypokinetic segments: Influence of tethering from adjacent segments. *Echocardiography.* 2002; 19:475–481.

46. Baer FM, Theissen P, Schneider CA, et al. Dobutamine magnetic resonance imaging predicts contractile recovery of chronically dysfunctional myocardium after successful revascularization. *J Am Coll Cardiol.* 1998; 31:1040–1048.

47. Bax JJ, de Roos A, van Der Wall EE. Assessment of myocardial viability by MRI. *J Magn Reson Imaging.* 1999; 10:418–422.

48. Ramani K, Judd RM, Holly TA, et al. Contrast magnetic resonance imaging in the assessment of myocardial viability in patients with stable coronary artery disease and left ventricular dysfunction. *Circulation.* 1998; 98:2687–2694.

49. Smedema JP, Snoep G, Van Kroonenburgh M, Eerens F. Left ventricular viability in a patient with heart failure due to left main stem stenosis, predicted by SPECT and gadolinium-enhanced magnetic resonance but not by dobutamine stress echocardiography. *Cardiovasc J S Afr.* 2006; 17:24–26.

50. Bucciarelli-Ducci C, Wu E, Lee DC, Holly TA, Klocke FJ, Bonow RO. Contrast-enhanced cardiac magnetic resonance in the evaluation of myocardial infarction and myocardial viability in patients with ischemic heart disease. *Curr Probl Cardiol.* 2006; 31:128–168.

51. Bello D, Shah DJ, Farah GM, et al. Gadolinium cardiovascular magnetic resonance predicts reversible myocardial dysfunction and remodeling in patients with heart failure undergoing beta-blocker therapy. *Circulation.* 2003; 108:1945–1953.

52. Selvanayagam JB, Kardos A, Francis JM, et al. Value of delayed-enhancement cardiovascular magnetic resonance imaging in predicting myocardial viability after surgical revascularization. *Circulation.* 2004; 110:1535–1541.

53. Bove CM, DiMaria JM, Voros S, Conaway MR, Kramer CM. Dobutamine response and myocardial infarct transmurality: Functional improvement after coronary artery bypass grafting—initial experience. *Radiology.* 2006; 240:835–841.

54. Gerber BL, Garot J, Bluemke DA, Wu KC, Lima JA. Accuracy of contrast-enhanced magnetic resonance imaging in predicting improvement of regional myocardial function in patients after acute myocardial infarction. *Circulation.* 2002; 106:1083–1089.

55. Motoyasu M, Sakuma H, Ichikawa Y, et al. Prediction of regional functional recovery after acute myocardial infarction with low dose dobutamine stress cine MR imaging and contrast enhanced MR imaging. *J Cardiovasc Magn Reson.* 2003; 5:563–574.

56. Ergun I, Keven K, Uruc I, et al. The safety of gadolinium in patients with stage 3 and 4 renal failure. *Nephrol Dial Transplant.* 2006; 21:697–700.

57. Mickleborough LL, Maruyama H, Takagi Y, Mohamed S, Sun Z, Ebisuzaki L. Results of revascularization in patients with severe left ventricular dysfunction. *Circulation.* 1995; 92:II73–II79.

58. Alderman EL, Fisher LD, Litwin P, et al. Results of coronary artery surgery in patients with poor left ventricular function (CASS). *Circulation.* 1983; 68:785–795.

59. Samady H, Elefteriades J, Abbott B, Mattera J, McPherson C, Wackers F. Failure to improve left ventricular function after coronary revascularization for ischemic cardiomyopathy is not associated with worse outcome. *Circulation.* 1999; 100:1298–1304.

60. Lapu-Bula R, Robert A, De Kock M, et al. Relation of exercise capacity to left ventricular systolic function and diastolic filling in idiopathic or ischemic dilated cardiomyopathy. *Am J Cardiol.* 1999; 83:728–734.

61. Franciosa JA, Park M, Levine TB. Lack of correlation between exercise capacity and indexes of resting left ventricular performance in heart failure. *Am J Cardiol.* 1981; 47:33–39.

62. Bax JJ, Poldermans D, Elhendy A, et al. Improvement of left ventricular ejection fraction, heart failure symptoms and prognosis after revascularization in patients with chronic coronary artery disease and viable myocardium detected by dobutamine stress echocardiography. *J Am Coll Cardiol.* 1999; 34:163–169.

63. Pagano D, Townend JN, Littler WA, Horton R, Camici PG, Bonser RS. Coronary artery bypass surgery as treatment for ischemic heart failure: The predictive value of viability assessment with quantitative positron emission tomography for symptomatic and functional outcome. *J Thorac Cardiovasc Surg.* 1998; 115:791–799.

5

Coronary CT Angiography

5.1   Basic Physics and the CT Camera

Kavitha M. Chinnaiyan, Laxmi S. Mehta, Ralph E. Gentry, and Gilbert L. Raff

Overivew of Computed Tomography

Dramatic improvements in multi-detector computed tomography (MDCT) technology over the last decade have vastly increased its clinical utility and popularity for cardiac imaging. Because of its easy acquisition, improved spatial and temporal resolution, and flexible interpretation in three dimensions, coronary CT angiography is now considered by some to be the new alternative to invasive angiography.

Evolution of CT Scanners

The basic principle of the CT scanner is the use of a thin, fan-shaped X-ray beam that passes through the body to a detector array, which then measures the degree of the X-ray transmission. This data is then digitized into picture elements called pixels. A pixel is a small region of a grid of the imaged object whose size depends on the size of each detector and its surrounding lead shielding (collimator). Various shades of gray are assigned to the pixels representing the imaged structures. This data is reconstructed into an image using a computer program based on mathematical back-calculation of the attenuation from the body ("algorithmic back-projection"). The anatomic image data can be displayed on computer workstations and can be flexibly sliced and rotated, and displayed in various two- and three-dimensional formats to aid in interpretation, which is critically important in the tortuous coronary circulation.

The first CT scanner was introduced for clinical use in 1973. Since then, the CT technology used for routine clinical diagnostic examinations has progressed through four generations of development. The first generation of CT scanners consisted of an X-ray tube that generated a thin "pencil beam" and a single detector. Both the X-ray tube and the detector moved as an assembly in a rectilinear path across the gantry. A series of 1-degree rotations-translations across a 180° arc were necessary to produce an image, resulting in long scan times. Scan time with the second-generation CT systems using a fan-shaped X-ray beam and a group of detectors (detector array) decreased scan times considerably. Third-generation systems use a fan-shaped X-ray beam and a detector array arranged in a curved arc rather than a straight line. This results in rotation of the X-ray tube/detector assembly around the patient, rather than a rectilinear path across the patient. Continuous rotation (the current third-generation) scanners were introduced to eliminate the problem of winding up of the high-tension cable from the high frequency generator that required stopping the gantry frame and reversing direction with each subsequent scan. Continuous rotation scanners use a large rotating ring that surrounds the gantry aperture (the slip ring) and eliminates the winding up of the cable. Electrical brushes convey electrical power and data to the components mounted on the rotating ring. The slip ring conveys scanning instructions from the host computer to the gantry components and may serve to facilitate image reconstruction by conveying information about measured attenuation data from the patient to the computer. The combination of rotation and movement of the patient produces a spiral or helical path of the X-ray tube with respect to the patient. This results in extremely fast scan times. The majority of medical CT scanners in use today, including all cardiac scanners, are third-generation spiral technology. Fourth-generation scanners consist of a fan-shaped X-ray beam with detectors forming a complete circle around the gantry in a ring configuration. In these scanners, the X-ray tube rotates while the detectors are stationary. Because the detectors completely surround the gantry, the number of detectors needed is large.

Multi-row detector scanners were introduced to decrease scan time without compromising anatomical data. These scanners consist of multiple parallel detector arrays and a thick X-ray beam. Each detector array is in turn composed of several hundred detectors arranged along a curved arc. MDCT scanners collect data from multiple anatomical slices in each rotation of the X-ray tube, leading to faster scan times because of wider coverage. Cardiac imaging became practical once breath-hold was reduced to 20 seconds or less (16-slice technology). This has been improved further by the wide availability of 64-slice scanners that have reduced breath-hold times to 15 seconds or less for most patients.

In the MDCT systems, an X-ray tube mounted on a rotating gantry generates the X-ray photons and an array of detectors is positioned to receive the photons after they "go through" the patient situated in the bore of the gantry. The number of X-ray photons can be increased by increasing the *tube current (mA)* via a tungsten filament, typically to allow better tissue penetration and diminished image noise in patients with higher body mass indices. With the MDCT systems, the gantry rotates continuously and the table moves the patient through the imaging plane at a set speed. *Scan pitch* is the relative speed of the gantry rotation table speed, and is important for cardiac gating in the helical mode.

$$Pitch = Table\ Speed/Collimator\ Width$$

Thus, the faster the table speed, the wider the slices. For high-resolution cardiac imaging, very thin axial slices are required, i.e., lower table speed. The disadvantage of a low table speed is higher radiation exposure. The fastest available rotation time for MDCT systems is 333 milliseconds. Spatial resolution can be preserved by increasing collimator coverage and consequent lowering of the pitch. In the 64-slice systems with 0.625 mm collimation and table feed of 3.8 mm per rotation with the tube current at 120 kV, pitch is equal to 0.1 with an average scan time of 6–10 seconds.

Spatial resolution is the ability of the system to effectively depict and reproduce fine details within an image. Spatial resolution is dependent on slice thickness as well as the reconstruction matrix. *Temporal resolution* is the amount of time taken to acquire necessary scan data to reconstruct an image (Figure 5.1). For multiscan CT, temporal resolution depends on the time taken by the scanner to complete one gantry rotation, which can be modified using partial scan or "half-scan" reconstruction techniques. Half-scan reconstruction uses scan data from a 180° (in reality, 210° when the fan beam width is considered) gantry rotation to generate a singe axial image. This results in improved temporal resolution, i.e., 60% of the rotation speed of the scanner.

Although development of 16- and 64-slice spiral CT systems has resulted in an *increase* in gantry rotation times (from 500 milliseconds to 330 milliseconds) and subsequent improved temporal resolution, the scanning algorithms of these systems display a nonlinear relationship with heart rate (Figure 5.2), making them sensitive to changes in heart rate during image acquisition. The 330 milliseconds per revolution rotation speed is close to the physical limits the components of the gantry assembly can endure. Because algorithmic back-projection requires only a half-scan (180° rotation) to produce a full image, the effective "shutter speed" of a 330-millisecond rotation scanner is approximately 165 milliseconds (Figures 5.3 and 5.4). This requires both heart rate

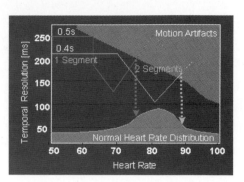
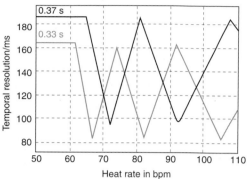

FIGURE 5.1 Effect of rotation speed on temporal resolution.
Courtesy of Siemens AG Medical Solutions, Forchheim and Erlangen, Germany.

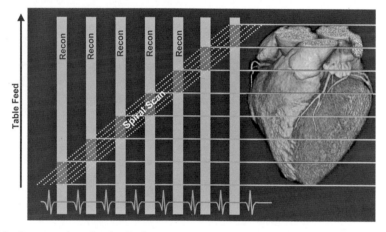

FIGURE 5.2 Scan speed synchronized to heart rate.
Courtesy of Siemens AG Medical Solutions, Forchheim and Erlangen, Germany.

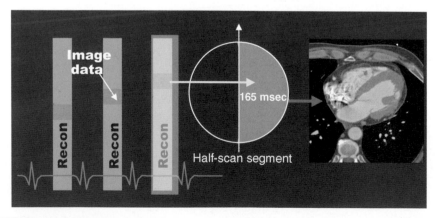

FIGURE 5.3 Single segment reconstruction.
Courtesy of Siemens AG Medical Solutions, Forchheim and Erlangen, Germany.

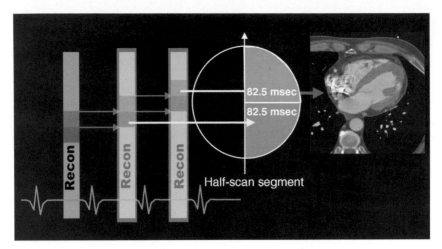

FIGURE 5.4 Multi-segment reconstruction.
Courtesy of Siemens AG Medical Solutions, Forchheim and Erlangen, Germany.

reduction (to 60–70 beats per minute) and heart rate stabilization to avoid image artifacts caused by motion (either blurring or "reconstruction" artifacts). Thus, in most patients, lowering of heart rates is achieved by pretreatment with beta-blocking drugs.

Dual-Source CT

The dual-source CT (DSCT) system is equipped with two X-ray tubes and two corresponding detectors mounted onto the gantry with an angular offset of 90°. One detector covers the entire scan field of view (50 cm), while the other detector covers a smaller, central field of view (26 cm). Each detector has 40 detector rows (32 central rows with 0.6 mm collimated slice width, and four outer rows with 1.2 mm collimated slice width). Two subsequent 32-slice readings with 0.6 mm collimated slice width are combined to one 64-slice projection with a sampling distance of 0.3 mm at the isocenter. Thus, 64 overlapping 0.6 mm slices per rotation are acquired, with a gantry rotation time of 0.33 seconds. The temporal resolution is either 83 milliseconds with a single R-R reconstruction, or 42 milliseconds with a segmented reconstruction algorithm combining data from two cardiac cycles. Dual-source CT enables reconstruction of cross-sectional images with a temporal resolution corresponding to one quarter of the gantry rotation time in the center of the gantry rotation, reducing the effective temporal resolution to approximately 83 milliseconds as of this writing. This generally permits artifact-free scanning without beta-blockers in most patients.

Image Formation

Cross-sectional images are obtained when the thin, fan-shaped X-ray beam passes through the body at many angles. The corresponding X-ray transmission measurements are collected by a detector array. Information entering the detector array and X-ray beam is collimated to produce thin sections while avoiding photon scatter. The data recorded by the detectors are digitized into picture elements (pixels) with dimensions that determine the effective resolution of the scanner. Thus, a scanner that produces pixels that are 0.6 mm by 0.6 mm will effectively produce resolution close to 0.6 mm in tissue. The third dimension, the thickness of the slices, creates a third side to the cube (a volume-element or voxel), which is incorporated into a three-dimensional dataset incorporating everything within the thorax, or other body parts within the field of view. It is important that the third dimension (slice thickness) be equivalent to the other dimension of the pixel (producing an isotropic volume element or voxel) that is the same on all three dimensions. This allows accurate rotation of the processed image without anatomic distortion (see below). Grayscale values for voxels in the reconstructed tomogram are defined with reference to the value for water, called CT numbers or Hounsfield units (HU). The grayscale information contained in each pixel is reconstructed according to the attenuation of the X-ray beam along its path using a standardized technique called algorithmic back-projection. This back-projection is further filtered mathematically to avoid sharp artifacts, resulting in a filtered back-projection. Once this data is reconstructed, it can be flexibly sampled retrospectively within any plane using the multi-planar reformat technique.

Differences in brightness of the image at different points will depend on physical density as well as the presence of atoms with a high difference in atomic number (for example, calcium, soft tissue, and water). The CT brightness of the image results from atoms absorbing (attenuating) the X-ray beam differently. Blood and soft tissue have similar densities and consist of similar proportions of the same atoms (hydrogen, carbon, and oxygen), whereas bone has an abundance of calcium and fat has abundant hydrogen. The higher the density of the constituent atoms, the brighter the structure on the CT images. Hence, calcium is bright white, air is black, and soft tissue (blood and muscle) is gray. Although non-contrast CT can readily distinguish blood from air, fat, and bone, it cannot distinguish blood easily from muscle or soft tissue. Because the lumen of the coronary arteries contains water-density blood adjacent to similar density muscle, in general the two cannot be distinguished on a non-contrast scan, whereas the high-density calcium is clearly visible. To distinguish blood from soft tissue (for example, lumen from wall of the coronary artery), injection of contrast is necessary. The absorption of the X-rays by calcium and iodine (elements of high atomic number) allows superb visualization of the lumen of the coronary arteries and coronary calcium as well, although calcium scoring must be done on a non-contrast scan. Hounsfield units may range from −1000 (air) through 0 (water) to +1000 (bone) because of differences in attenuation of X-ray. Coronary calcium caused by atherosclerosis generally measures 130–600 HU. Metal found in valves, wires, stents, and surgical clips can measure +1000 HU or greater.

Prospective Versus Retrospective Gating

Historically, CT imaging of the heart has been challenging, primarily because of continuous motion. The development of electrocardiograph (ECG)-synchronized MDCT scanning and reconstruction techniques now enables fast volume coverage as well as high spatial and temporal resolution. In addition, appropriate collimation size and scan acquisition speed should be chosen to minimize motion artifacts. Collimation size for CT calcium scoring as well as coronary angiography is 0.6–3 mm, with acquisition time of 50–250 milliseconds per image. However, this "ultra-fast" speed is not enough to eliminate cardiac motion. Hence, cardiac or ECG triggering is necessary to minimize cardiac and coronary motion during scan acquisition and to improve image quality. Cardiac motion is lower by nearly 30 milliseconds in early diastole, and thus, this interval is most favorable to obtain adequate images.

Multi-detector CT systems can operate in two modes of scanning: prospective triggered or retrospective gating. In the prospective triggered mode (sequential), a signal is derived from the R wave of the patient's ECG and using this "trigger," scanning is performed over a finite period of the R-R interval, usually in ventricular diastole (period of the least cardiac motion) (Figure 5.5). This mode is used in calcium scoring protocols in most centers. By prospectively acquiring images with a "step and shoot" approach during a finite period, radiation exposure

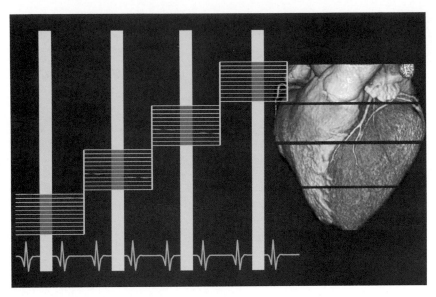

FIGURE 5.5 Prospective electrocardiographic triggering.
Courtesy of Siemens AG Medical Solutions, Forchheim and Erlangen, Germany.

is reduced. In this mode, 16 or 64 simultaneous data channels of image information can be acquired in the 16- or 64-slice scanner. Larger volumes of coverage per rotation with a 64-slice scanner compared to a 16-slice scanner (40 mm versus 20 mm) results in improved 3D modeling with short imaging times. The drawbacks of this type of gating include high sensitivity to cardiac motion artifacts and image misregistration, particularly in patients with arrhythmias. In the retrospective gating mode (helical), continuous radiation is applied and large volumes (hundreds to thousands) of images are obtained (Figure 5.6). The images are then

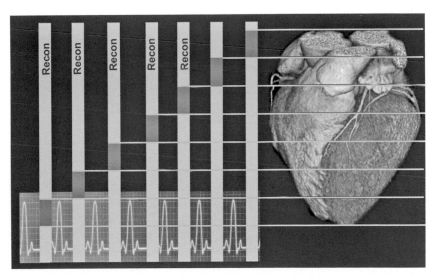

FIGURE 5.6 Retrospective electrocardiographic triggering.
Courtesy of Siemens AG Medical Solutions, Forchheim and Erlangen, Germany.

retrospectively aligned to the ECG tracing, and for static images, image reconstruction is usually performed at 60%–65% of the cardiac cycle. Current MDCT systems have an X-ray gantry rotation time of 500 milliseconds or less, the fastest being 333 milliseconds or less. Thus, with faster heart rates, as in systole or with premature atrial contractions, resulting motion artifacts distort final images, and multiple data sets would have to be examined for the reconstruction demonstrating the least cardiac motion and artifacts.

Relative timing and fixed timing are two types of retrospective ECG gating. *Relative timing* involves reconstructing the images at a specific percentage of the R-R interval. Typical reconstruction intervals include 65% of the R-R interval (mid-diastole) and 35% of the R-R interval (end-systole). Although the left coronary system is frequently analyzed at end-diastole, this may not be adequate for the right coronary artery, which is frequently found to have coronary motion artifact. Atrial fibrillation, ectopic beats, or variation in the heart rate during the scan affect image quality and transaxial continuity of the images when relative timing reconstruction methods are used. *Fixed timing* is based on determining a fixed duration of time after each R wave that the images will be reconstructed. This is most helpful in patients with faster heart rates and irregular heart rates, such as atrial fibrillation.

Contrast Injection

The goal of injection of contrast material is to increase the contrast between the coronary arteries and the surrounding structures. Injection of contrast material leads to an increase in Hounsfield units of the target structure (coronary arteries). Factors to consider with regard to contrast injection are the scan delay time (also known as the circulation time) and the method of injection.

Scan delay time is the time required for the contrast to travel from the site of injection (usually an antecubital vein) to the proximal aorta. Several factors influence this time, including cardiac output, venous anatomy, and age. Scan delay time is used in two different forms. One method uses a test bolus of 10–15 mL of contrast material injected at a rate of 3–5 mL per second, and the scan delay time is measured with serial scanning of the same slice (typically the proximal aorta) to obtain the peak enhancement time (typically 120 HU) through a time density curve analysis (typically 10–12 seconds). The care bolus is then injected accordingly. The other method is to use an automatic bolus-triggering technique. With this method, the first monitoring scan is obtained 10–12 seconds after beginning the contrast injection, and when the HU reaches 120 HU, coronary angiographic imaging is automatically activated.

The doses of the contrast depend on not only the desired enhancement level (HU), but also the patient size and scan time. Typically, 70–120 mL of contrast agent at a rate of 5 mL per second followed by saline injection is used at our institution. For the "triple rule-out" protocol, the injection rate is 5 mL per second for the first 100 mL, followed by 3 mL per second for the last 20 mL (total contrast volume of 120 mL).

Image Reconstruction

The raw data is post-processed with specific CT reconstruction algorithms, the filtered back-projection being the most widely recognized and used method. During simple back-projection the attenuation value for each ray spreads across similar paths within the image, resulting in a blurred image. Mathematical reconstruction filters, also known as *kernels,* are used to smoothen or sharpen the images by filtering the raw data, also known as the convolution technique. Smooth kernel images have better contrast detail, lower noise level, and poorer spatial resolution compared to sharp kernel images. Sharp kernel images have better spatial resolution, higher noise level, and better edge definition, and therefore are frequently used in the evaluation of coronary artery stents or segments with dense calcification. Images are typically reconstructed with a slice thickness of 0.6–0.75 mm and 50% overlap of consecutive transaxial slices. In obese patients, the slice thickness is increased to 1 mm in order to reduce image noise from soft tissue attenuation.

Post-Processing Techniques

Several different reconstruction techniques are employed in CT angiography image analysis. Image post-processing involves reformatting the original CT images, volume- and surface-rendered displays, and physiologic imaging analysis. It is important to remember that reformatting does not alter the CT voxels in any way. This process uses the voxels in off-axis views and displays the images produced from the original reconstruction in different orientations. Standard methods include sagittal, coronal, oblique, and curved reformatting. Other reformatting techniques frequently used in cardiac imaging include volume rendering technique (VRT), maximum intensity projection (MIP), and multiplanar reformatting (MPR). Although three-dimensional displays (VRT) that emulate gross anatomy are visually captivating, they are rarely used for assessment of luminal stenoses. Two-dimensional reconstructed images (MIP and MPR) that emulate fluoroscopic projections are predominately used for image analysis.

The **volume rendering** technique (VRT) provides a three-dimensional depiction of the heart and is based on depicting pixels above a certain HU threshold. Pixels with an HU below the set value will be removed and the remaining pixels are assigned an HU value by the computer. VRT images provide a volume of anatomic data in various cut planes, allowing visualization of the anatomic course of the vessels. Measurement of luminal stenosis can be performed and the lumen can be analyzed in various angles. A significant drawback is the loss of fine detail in smaller vessels caused by a "smoothing" effect that is characteristic of this reconstruction technique, and both calcium and intravascular contrast remain bright since their HU is well above the cutoff value. Consequently, plaque visualization is inadequate with this reconstruction technique. VRT images are particularly useful in identification of coronary artery bypass grafts and intra-myocardial bridging of coronary arteries.

The **maximal intensity projection** (MIP) post-processing technique is the most frequently used reconstruction method for analysis of CT angiography images. The MIP images project the brightest pixel (highest value) at each point in the visualized plane, resulting in an image similar to fluoroscopic angiography. Cross-sectional images are produced by assigning each pixel a grayscale value that correlates with the attenuation of the structure. Unfortunately, low attenuating structures are masked by high attenuation structures, so 3D data is not provided in areas of overlapping structures with various densities. Dense structures such as calcium and coronary stents are bright and hinder accurate assessment of underlying luminal stenoses. Contrast-enhanced lumen can be distinguished from calcium and coronary stents by differences in "brightness" between these structures. Noncalcified ("soft") plaque can also be assessed with MIP techniques, since the lower density structures (thrombus, fibrotic tissue) appear as filling defects within the lumen. MIP images allow visualization of distal vessels and small caliber vessels without the smoothing effect seen on VRT images. Reconstruction of images throughout the cardiac cycle also allows visualization of ventricular function using four-dimensional software programs.

The MPR post-processing technique is also known as the **curved surface reformation technique.** This method allows visualization of the entire coronary tree in one view by following the course of the vessel. The centerline of the coronary artery is tracked and the computer provides cross-sectional cuts of the artery that are orthogonal to the centerline. MPR has been shown to have a high sensitivity and specificity. Many centers prefer this method of image analysis since it can be performed relatively quickly and is reproducible without manual segmentation of the entire coronary tree. Limitations of this method include computer-generated stenoses since the true centerline may be questionable, visualization of only one vessel at a time, and the requirement that side branches be separately evaluated as they are not depicted as part of the main artery. In addition, motion artifacts and respiration artifacts are not identifiable with MPR.

CT Artifacts

Artifacts can significantly affect image quality and sometimes make images impossible to interpret. Artifacts can be separated into three categories: physics-based, patient-based, and scanner-based.

Physics-Based Artifacts

Beam hardening artifact is the increase in the mean energy of the X-ray beam as it passes through the tissue. This is a result of dense tissues such as calcium preferentially absorbing the lower energy photons so that the detectors capture only photons with a higher mean energy. Beams passing through the center of the tissue are affected by beam hardening more than those in the peripheral tissue, resulting in an image with a cup-like contour. Streaks or dark bands may also be seen between dense objects as a result of beam hardening artifact. Beam hardening artifact may be minimized with implementation of filtration, calibration correction, and beam hardening correction software.

Partial volume effect is the averaging of all densities within a voxel. Calcium deposits have a higher density than other structures, so calcium overshadows the other tissues. As a result, the voxel may be disproportionately bright because of the presence of even a small degree of calcium, known as the "blooming" artifact. Partial volume artifacts manifest as objects with blurry margins as a result of peripheral dense objects projecting into the pathway of a wide X-ray beam. This can be avoided by obtaining thinner slices at the expense of increased image noise.

Patient-Based Artifacts

Motion artifacts can occur as a result of respiratory motion, movement on the table, and coronary motion artifact. The resultant images have ***misregistration*** artifact with the appearance of streaks within the image (Figure 5.7). Also, blurring of the tissue contours can occur.

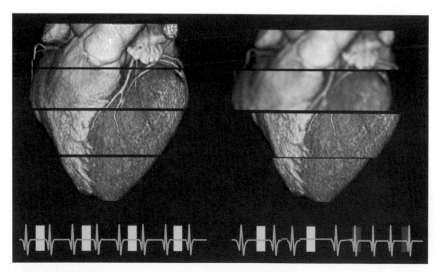

FIGURE 5.7 Misregistration artifact.
Courtesy of Siemens AG Medical Solutions, Forchheim and Erlangen, Germany.

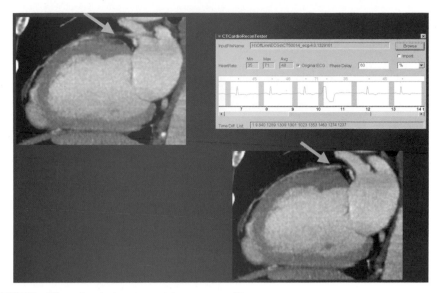

FIGURE 5.8   Effect of a single extra-systole on scan quality.
Courtesy of Siemens AG Medical Solutions, Forchheim and Erlangen, Germany.

Respiratory and patient motion may be minimized with thorough coaching of the patient prior to the scan. Coronary artery motion artifact is most frequently seen in the mid right coronary artery, as this segment is perpendicular to the transverse slices obtained in the raw data. With motion of the vessel, misregistration in consecutive slices can be seen in the coronal view. Arrhythmias (atrial fibrillation, ectopic beats, or change in heart rhythm during the scan) also cause misregistration artifacts (Figures 5.8 and 5.9). Image reconstructions with multiple phases throughout the cardiac cycle allow segmental visualization of the artery and minimize motion artifacts.

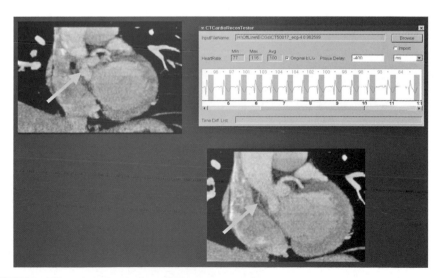

FIGURE 5.9   Effect of an irregular heart rhythm on scan quality.
Courtesy of Siemens AG Medical Solutions, Forchheim and Erlangen, Germany.

Metallic structures within the heart (coronary stents, pacing wires, mechanical prosthetic valves) create severe *streaking* artifacts. The metal density exceeds the computer-generated normal density range. Metallic objects may also result in beam hardening and partial volume artifacts, which hinder adequate visualization (for example, arterial lumen within the struts of a stent). Using thinner slices during image acquisition can minimize metallic partial volume artifacts. In addition, increasing the tube current (mA) during acquisition may allow the X-ray beam to penetrate the object better. Reconstructing images with a sharper (harder) kernel may also allow better evaluation of intracoronary stents.

Out of field artifact occurs when a portion of the patient's body or other dense structures (for example, an intravenous tube with contrast material) outside of the scan field of view is present during image acquisition. The X-ray beam passes through this structure and the resultant beam is subject to attenuation and beam hardening. This artifact can be avoided by positioning the patient so that structures (arms, intravenous tubing) are out of the path of the X-ray beam.

Scanner-Based Artifacts

Ring artifact occurs when one of the detectors on a third-generation scanner is not calibrated. Thus, the detector provides an abnormal reading at each angle around the patient. Faulty detectors can be recognized on the localizer image as a straight line down the length of the image, indicating that the detector needs to be recalibrated or repaired. *Tube arching* is another form of scanner-based artifact that occurs when the scanner is older. The resultant artifact can vary in severity from minor streaks in the image to loss of the entire image.

Cone beam artifacts are more apparent with an increasing number of detector rows as the X-ray beam becomes cone-shaped rather than fan-shaped with the wider collimation. This artifact gives a "star-like" appearance to the peripheral tissues in the image. The inner detector rows have less apparent star-like artifact, as they are closer to the imaging plane as opposed to the outer detector rows.

Another artifact that is very rare is the *stair step* artifact. This artifact occurs at the edges of the structures when nonoverlapping reconstruction intervals are used on the earlier generation CT scanners.

Radiation Dose

Radiation dose from CT scans is among the highest in diagnostic radiology. Although ionizing radiation from natural sources constitutes daily life, the potential risk of the excessively high radiation from CT scan procedures should be weighed against potential benefits. Diagnostic medical radiation exposures consist of up to half of the radiation exposure to the population. The effective dose (E) (introduced in 1975 to assess effects of radiation from partial body irradiations compared to whole-body irradiations) for an X-ray–based test is the weighted sum of the doses to a number of body tissues. The weighting factor for each tissue depends on its relative sensitivity to radiation-induced cancer or severe hereditary defects attributed to genetic mutations. Effective dose is a standard measure that therefore allows comparison of medical and nonmedical exposures. The unit for the effective dose is sievert (Sv): 100 mrem = 1 mSv. Several methods exist for calculation of the effective dose. The average annual background radiation in the United States is about 300 mrem (3 mSv).

E from a CT examination can be calculated from radiation exposure measured through several different methods. It can also be estimated from dose length product (DLP) displayed by the CT scanner. DLP is an indication of the integrated radiation dose of the entire examination and incorporates the scan width (DLP = $CTDI_{vol}$ × scan length). Most contemporary CT scanners display $CTDI_{vol}$. Additionally, a rough estimate of E is obtained by multiplying DLP by a conversion factor (k). K values have been published for the head, neck, abdomen, and pelvis.

Sources of error in estimating E in CT examinations include the following:

1. Body size. Patients who are larger than ideal size absorb more radiation and to different organs than usually estimated. Also, the weighting factor of dosage depth does not take into consideration patient size.
2. Sex differences. Female breasts have a higher sensitivity to the effects of radiation than those of the male. Radiation scatter differs among gonads depending on the part of the body undergoing the CT examination.
3. Body position. CT examination of the chest with the patient in the supine position is associated with a lower effective dose than the same examination in the prone position because of issues related to depth of X-ray penetration.
4. Individual variation from average models. Individual organ sensitivity may vary from idealized models because of age, organ size, or location.
5. Errors in exposure dose measurements.

Although the risk of radiation-induced cancer in any one person is small (increase in the possibility of fatal cancer of one chance in 2000), this small increase in radiation risk for one person can become a major public health concern if large numbers of the population undergo CT scans for purposes of screening. Thus, dose reduction and avoidance is of paramount importance, and is dependent on the protocol used.

Variables that affect radiation dose in clinical coronary CT angiography:

1. Scan length (in cm). The scan region of the patient's body in the scanner's ***field of view*** (FOV) is variable in the Z direction and affects absorption of the X-ray photons by a value of the cube of the entire length. Thus, proper attention to length is necessary. Instead of rigidly scanning from carina to diaphragm (frequently recommended by scanner manufacturers), length may be determined by examination of the calcium scan to set the upper limit above the apex of the left anterior descending artery (LAD) (the highest artery) to the bottom of the posterior descending artery (PDA). While using this method, it is vital that the breath-hold is to the same depth as the "scout" calcium score in order to avoid "cutting off" of the arteries. Understandably, both scan length and scan time are affected by the "triple rule-out" protocol to evaluate for coronary artery disease, pulmonary embolism, and aortic dissection simultaneously. Because of the consequent steep increase in radiation exposure, there must be a strong clinical rationale to use this protocol.
2. Scan time (in seconds). Scan duration is a variable affected by the table pitch in helical scans, which is in turn affected by the number of slices in the scanner, the size of the detector array, and the use of additional modalities such as dual source tubes. Scan time is also affected by scan length as well as slice thickness, with an increase in slice thickness leading to faster pitch, shorter time, and lower radiation dose. Radiation dose is directly proportional to the duration of the scan.
3. Tube amperage (mA). Tube mA is a variable setting that affects the number of photons generated and so affects image signal/noise. Radiation dose is approximately directly proportional to mA, and customarily, amperage can be adjusted for body mass and configuration, since patients with higher mass will experience higher photon scatters and higher noise. Failure to adjust mA downward for thin patients will result in unnecessary radiation.
4. Tube voltage [kV(p)]. Tube kV(p) determines peak photon energy and affects image contrast. Although adjustment of mA for body mass index is generally used, recent data suggest a 20% reduction in radiation dose by decreasing the kV(p) in thin patients, with 100 kV(p) being advocated by some experts. Radiation dose is proportional approximately to the square of the tube voltage.

5. Electrocardiographic pulsing. Current generation scanners are capable of varying tube output in synchrony to the patient's electrocardiogram, a process called "dose modulation." This is done to reduce radiation during the most dynamic phases of the cardiac cycle. The ideal "pulsing window" is as short as possible. This becomes a complex decision, as there is a trade-off between pulse window width, heart rate, and scanner type. The use of ECG pulsing can decrease radiation dose by 50% or more and is generally recommended unless other parameters threaten image quality (such as irregular heart rate).

6. Patient body mass. In general, patients with a body mass index greater than 30 are exposed to higher than usual radiation doses because of scatter and the requirement for higher tube output. This increased risk of radiation exposure should be taken into the risk/benefit decision, particularly since image quality can be seriously compromised without these adjustments to scanning parameters.

7. Scanner type. In general, increasing the number of detector rows and reducing detector size tends to increase the radiation dose. This is the result of the greater surface area of lead collimators (which can only be so thin while still being effective), which may be balanced against reduced scan times. Thus, the end result is complex. The complexity of these results is compounded by dual source scanners, which have two X-ray sources and detector rings operating during the scan time, but have a reduced scan time and heart-rate variable pitch. Theoretically, dual source scanners reduce scan time because their faster temporal resolution allows imaging faster heart rates (thereby reducing diastolic time). However, in practical experience, the higher temporal resolution is offset by the need for wider pulsing windows at higher heart rates.

8. Prospective versus retrospective gating. Retrospective gating is most widely used, because variable reconstruction windows have typically been necessary. However, because tube output is "on" throughout the cardiac cycle (albeit not constant with ECG pulsing), this results in longer effective scan time. Theoretically, in patients with slow and very steady heart rates, extremely low radiation dose can be achieved by prospective or sequential scanning with tube output "on" only during a narrow ECG window.

9. Noise. Noise is the standard deviation of pixel values measured within a uniform region of interest in the image (expressed in Hounsfield units). Noise is a quantitative measure of the amount of statistical variation in the image, and depends on the number of X-ray photons reaching the detector, electronic noise of the system, and the reconstruction kernel. In cardiac multi-detector row CT, radiation dose is increased without decreasing the noise with an improvement in temporal resolution.

Summary

Cardiac CT is complex, with challenges posed by several patient factors (cardiac motion, heart rate and rhythm variability, body mass index) and technical factors (scanner type and properties). These factors are essential to understand in order to obtain images that provide adequate information for diagnosis and subsequent treatment of cardiac disease.

REFERENCES

1. Nielson C, Kaiser DA, Fermano PA. *The CT Registry Review Program 2003*. Clifton, New Jersey: Medical Imaging Consultants, Inc.; 2003.
2. Budoff MJ. Computed tomography. In: Budoff MJ, Shinbane JS, eds. *Cardiac CT Imaging: Diagnosis of Cardiovascular Disease*. London: Springer-Verlag Limited; 2006:1–18, 41–66.
3. Kachelriess M, Ulzheimer S, Kalender WA. ECG-correlated image reconstruction from subsecond multi-slice spiral CT scans of the heart. *Med Phys*. 2000; 27:1881–1902.
4. Cody DD. AAPM/RSNA physics tutorial for residents: Topics in CT. Image processing in CT. *Radiographics*. 2002; 22:1255–1268.

5. Ohnesorge B, Flohr T, Becker C, et al. Cardiac imaging by means of electrocardiographically gated multisection spiral CT: Initial experience. *Radiology.* 2000; 217:564–571.

6. Achenbach S, Ulzheimer S, Baum U, et al. Noninvasive coronary angiography by retrospectively ECG-gated multislice spiral CT. *Circulation.* 2000; 102:2823–2828.

7. Giesler T, Baum U, Ropers D, Goldstein JA. Noninvasive visualization of coronary arteries using contrast-enhanced multidetector CT: Influence of heart rate on image quality and stenosis detection. *Am J Roentgenol.* 2002; 179:911–916.

8. Achenbach S, Ropers D, Kuettner A, et al. Contrast-enhanced coronary artery visualization by dual-source computed tomography: Initial experience. *Eur J Rad.* 2006; 57:331–335.

9. Raff GL, Gallagher MJ, O'Neill WW, Goldstein JA. Diagnostic accuracy of noninvasive coronary angiography using 64-slice spiral computed tomography. *J Am Coll Cardiol.* 2005; 46:552–557.

10. Sato T, Anno H, Kondo T, et al. Applicability of ECG-gated multislice helical CT to patients with atrial fibrillation. *Circ J.* 2005; 69:1068–1073.

11. Rubin GD, Dake MD, Napel S, et al. Spiral CT of renal artery stenosis: Comparison of three-dimensional rendering techniques. *Radiology.* 1994; 190:181–189.

12. Mao S, Takasu J, Child J, et al. Comparison of LV mass and volume measurements derived from electron beam tomography using cine imaging and angiographic imaging. *Int J Cardiovasc Imaging.* 2003; 19(5):439–445.

13. Schoepf JJ, Becker CB, Ohnesorge BM, et al. CT of coronary artery disease. *Radiology.* 2004; 232:18–37.

14. Kopp AF, Kuttner A, Trabold T, et al. Multislice CT in cardiac and coronary angiography. *Br J Radiol.* 2004; 77:87–97.

15. Achenbach S, Moshage W, Ropers D, Bachmann K. Curved multiplanar reconstructions for the evaluation of contrast-enhanced electron beam CT of the coronary arteries. *Am J Roentgenol.* 1998; 170:895–899.

16. Gaspar T, Halon DA, Lewis BS, et al. Diagnosis of coronary in-stent restenosis with multidetector row spiral computed tomography. *J Am Coll Cardiol.* 2005; 46(8):1573–1579.

17. Bae KT, Hong C, Whiting BR. Radiation dose in multidetector row computed tomography cardiac imaging. *J Magn Reson Imaging.* 2004; 19:859–863.

18. ICRP. *Recommendations of the International Commission on Radiological Protection.* Oxford: ICRP; 1991.

19. Mayo JR, Aldrich J, Muller NL. Radiation exposure at chest CT: A statement of the Fletschner Society. *Radiology.* 2003; 228:15–21.

20. Primak AN, McCollough CH, Brueswitz MR, et al. Relationship between noise, dose, and pitch in cardiac multidetector row CT. *Radiographics.* 2006; 26:1785–1794.

21. Morin RL, Gerber TC, McCollough CH. Radiation dose in computed tomography of the heart. *Circulation.* 2003; 107:917–922.

5.2   Clinical Examples and Scenarios

Kavitha M. Chinnaiyan and Laxmi S. Mehta

CASE 1

LAD Disease With Cardiac Catheterization Correlation

A 58-year-old woman with hyperlipidemia, hypertension, family history of premature coronary artery disease (CAD), and morbid obesity presents with chest pain of 3 weeks' duration. This pain is described as a left-sided chest pressure radiating to the left arm, shoulder, and jaw of moderate intensity and associated with diaphoresis and shortness of breath. These episodes occur with minimal exertion and resolve with resting. She undergoes a dipyridamole-induced stress myocardial perfusion imaging test that does not reveal perfusion defects. She is referred for coronary CT angiography.

Coronary CT angiography (CTA) reveals a high calcium score (246 Agatston units). In the mid-segment of the LAD, severe (nearly 80%) stenosis is appreciated (**Figures C1.1 and C1.2**). The patient subsequently undergoes cardiac catheterization and coronary angiography.

Coronary angiography (**Figures C1.3 and C1.4**) confirms severe concentric stenosis of the mid LAD (**Cine C1.1 and C1.2**). Percutaneous intervention is performed with placement of a drug-eluting stent and a decrease of the lesion from a severity of 80% to 0%, with excellent final anatomic results and no complications. She returns for follow-up 3 weeks later with a significant improvement in symptoms and resolution of chest pain.

Video Clips: C1.1 and C1.2 Coronary angiography of the left coronary system.

FIGURE C1.1 Coronary CT angiogram, foot (axial) view demonstrates the left main trifurcating into the LAD, ramus, and circumflex arteries. Dense calcification is appreciated at the origin of the left main and distal left main extending to the trifurcation. The mid-LAD displays severe narrowing (*arrow*). LAD, left anterior descending artery.

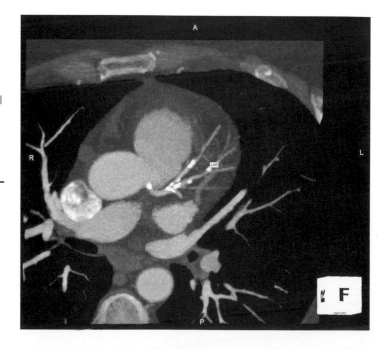

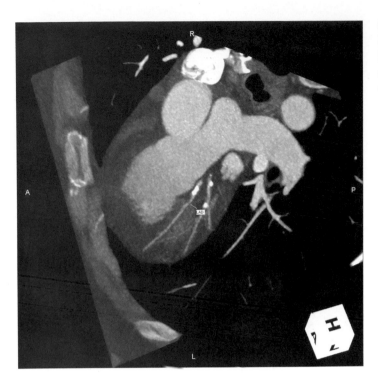

FIGURE C1.2 CT angiogram with LAD rotated anteriorly. The LAD lesion is visualized well. LAD, left anterior descending artery.

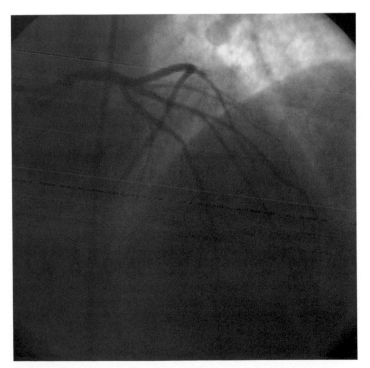

FIGURES C1.3 and C1.4 Coronary angiography of the left coronary system, right anterior oblique cranial view. (*continued*)

FIGURES C1.3 and C1.4 *(continued)*

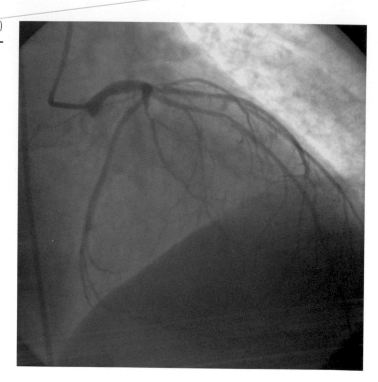

CASE 2

Effect of Overlying Calcium—Intravascular Ultrasound Correlation

A 69-year-old woman with hypertension and hyperlipidemia presents with palpitations of 2 months' duration. She reports that these episodes occur with her regular water exercises and are associated with symptoms of dyspnea, lasting a few minutes each time. There are no episodes at rest. She undergoes an exercise myocardial perfusion imaging study. At stage II of the Bruce protocol, she is found to have multiple premature ventricular beats and a six-beat salvo of nonsustained ventricular tachycardia at a rate of 150 beats per minute. The test is terminated. The perfusion imaging study is negative at the low workload. She is referred for coronary CT angiography for evaluation of a possible ischemic substrate for the arrhythmia.

Calcium score on CTA is high, with dense calcification present in the LAD. The ostial LAD is obscured by calcified plaque, and luminal stenosis is thought to be 40%–50% in severity (**Figures C2.1 and C2.2**). However, because of difficulty in accurate interpretation, the patient undergoes coronary angiography and intravascular ultrasound (IVUS) for further characterization of the LAD lesion.

Coronary angiography and intravascular ultrasound reveal mild disease in this segment. The patient is reassured and started on beta-blocker therapy for palpitations.

See Cine C2.1: Intravascular ultrasound of proximal left anterior descending artery.

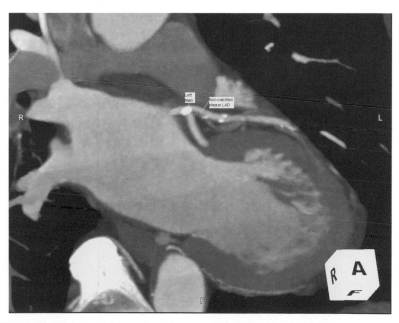

FIGURE C2.1   CT angiogram, right anterior oblique caudal view. This clearly demonstrates calcified plaque in the left main and LAD with non-calcified plaque at the ostial LAD. LAD, left anterior descending artery.

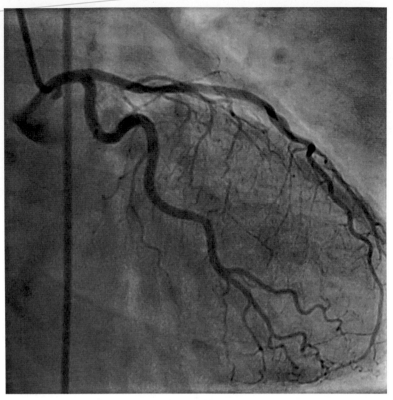

FIGURE C2.2   Coronary angiography, right anterior oblique caudal view reveals only mild disease in corresponding areas.

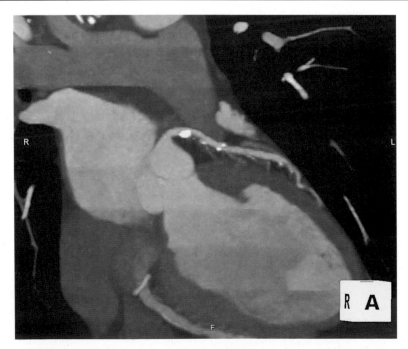

FIGURE C2.3   CT angiogram, right anterior oblique cranial view.

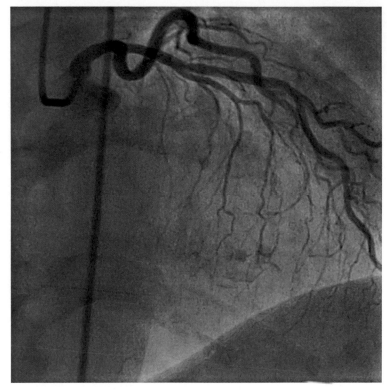

FIGURE C2.4   Coronary angiography, right anterior oblique cranial view.

Patent Intracoronary Stent

A 40-year-old male with hypertension and recent inferior myocardial infarction treated with primary angioplasty of the right coronary artery presents with recurrent chest pain radiating to the back. An urgent "triple-rule out" was ordered to evaluate for aortic dissection, an acute pulmonary embolism, or recurrent coronary artery disease. CT was negative for acute pulmonary embolism or aortic dissection.

Coronary CTA reveals a patent stent in the mid-right coronary artery (RCA). Distal to the stent, there is mild atherosclerotic disease with a severity of 20%–25% (**Figures C3.1 and C3.2**). The patient is medically treated and discharged in stable condition.

FIGURE C3.1 CT angiogram, anterior view. This displays the stent in the mid-RCA. Contrast is seen within the stent, indicative of a patent stent. RCA, right coronary artery.

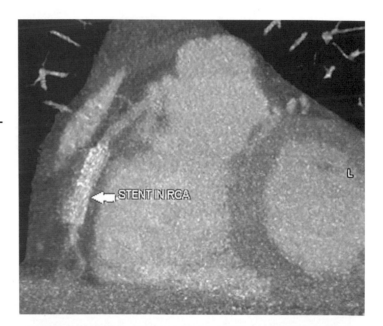

FIGURE C3.2 CT angiogram, foot (axial) view. The stent is seen end-on, with contrast visible within.

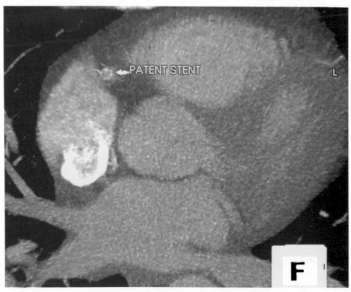

CASE 4

Three-Vessel Disease With Cardiac Catheterization Correlation

A 60-year-old woman with hypertension and atypical chest pain undergoes a stress myocardial perfusion imaging study. The myocardial perfusion image (MPI) reveals inducible perfusion defect involving the apex and the inferoapical area. The patient then undergoes a CTA to delineate the underlying coronary anatomy.

On CTA, calcium score is elevated at 117 Agatston units. Severe (greater than 70%) disease is appreciated in the proximal LAD, the first obtuse marginal branch of the left circumflex artery, and the distal right coronary artery (**Figures C4.1 and C4.2**).

Cardiac catheterization is then performed based on the findings on CTA. The LAD has a proximal 80% stenosis and severe disease at the ostium and proximal segment of the ramus (**Figures C4.3 and C4.4**) (**Cine C4.1 and C4.2**). The proximal circumflex artery also reveals significant disease. Multiple views are obtained of the right PDA when the lesion described on CTA is not seen in the traditional right anterior oblique (RAO) view (**Cine C4.3**). In the left anterior oblique (LAO) projection, a long, severe stenosis is observed in the proximal segment of the PDA (**Cine C4.4 and C4.5**).

The patient is referred for coronary artery bypass surgery, and undergoes grafting of the LAD with a left internal mammary artery (LIMA) graft and saphenous vein grafts to the ramus, PDA, and distal RCA. She remains clinically stable and asymptomatic.

Video Clips: C4.1 Video of the left coronary system, left anterior oblique cranial view; **C4.2** Video of the left coronary system, left anterior oblique caudal view; **C4.3** Video of the right coronary artery, right anterior oblique caudal view; **C4.4** Video of the right coronary artery, left anterior oblique caudal view; **C4.5** Video of the right coronary artery, right anterior oblique cranial view.

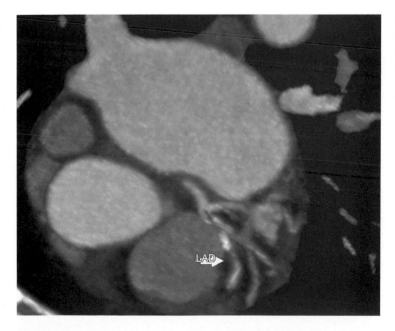

FIGURE C4.1 Left anterior oblique view of the LAD. Severe disease is noted in the proximal segment (*arrow*). LAD, left anterior desending artery.

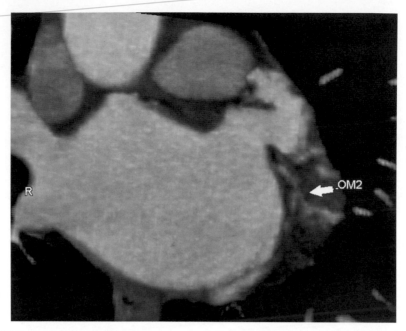

FIGURE C4.2 Axial view of the left coronary system; the image is "tilted" to view the left circumflex artery. Severe stenosis of the obtuse marginal branch is noted. OM2, Second Obtuse Marginal branch.

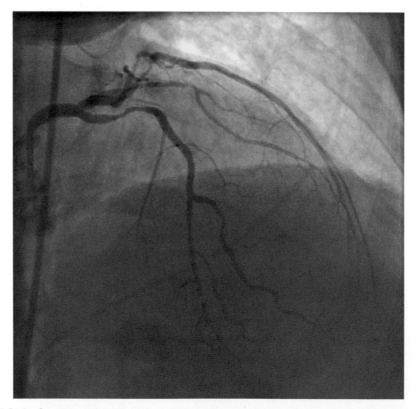

FIGURE C4.3 Coronary angiography, left coronary system.

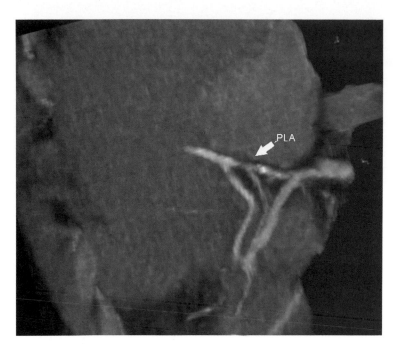

FIGURE C4.4   Axial view of the distal right coronary artery, demonstrating severe disease (*arrow*). PLA, Posterolateral artery.

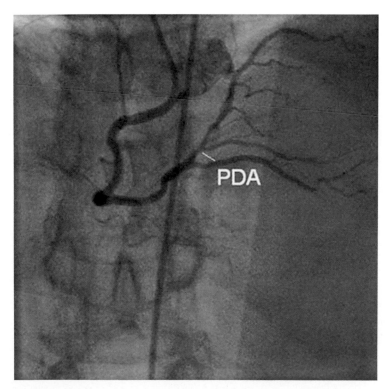

FIGURE C4.5   Coronary angiography of the right coronary artery, right anterior oblique cranial view. PDA, posterior descending artery.

CASE 5

Effect of High Calcium Score and Inaccuracy of Resultant Interpretation

An 83-year-old woman presents with atypical chest pain for which she undergoes a stress myocardial perfusion imaging study. The perfusion images reveal an anteroapical fixed defect with some reversibility (**Figures C5.1–C5.3**). After much discussion, the patient refuses a cardiac catheterization for further evaluation and opts for coronary CT angiogram instead.

On CTA, the calcium score is elevated at 1922 units. Large, dense calcified plaques obscure the left main, LAD, and circumflex arteries (**Figures C5.4 and C5.5**). The distal LAD is thought to be sub-totally or totally occluded. The RCA also reveals moderate calcification (**Figure C5.6**). Accurate interpretation of underlying stenosis is not possible and the patient is referred for cardiac catheterization.

On coronary angiography, the lumen of the left main shows mild disease, and the disease in the proximal LAD and circumflex is 40%–50% in severity (**Cine C5.1–C5.3**). The distal LAD is occluded. The RCA demonstrates mild luminal irregularities (**Cine C5.4**). The patient is started on medical therapy.

Video Clips: C5.1 Cineangiography, left coronary system, left anterior oblique caudal view; **C5.2** Cineangiography, left coronary system, right anterior oblique caudal view; **C5.3** Cineangiography, left coronary system, right anterior oblique cranial view; **C5.4** Cineangiography, right coronary artery, left anterior oblique cranial view.

FIGURE C5.1 CT angiogram: In this left anterior oblique caudal view of the left anterior descending artery (LAD), severe calcification is seen throughout the course of the vessel. The distal LAD is not visualized well.

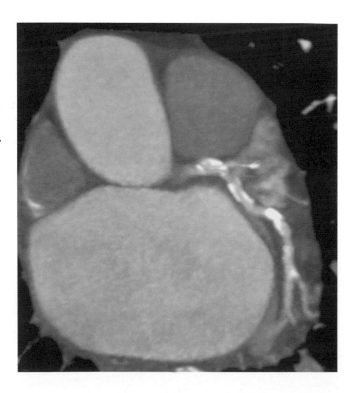

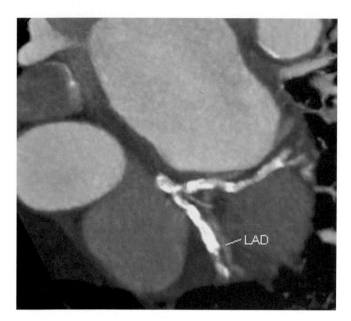

FIGURE C5.2 CT angiogram: In this left anterior oblique cranial view, severe disease is visualized in the LAD (*arrow*). LAD, left anterior descending artery.

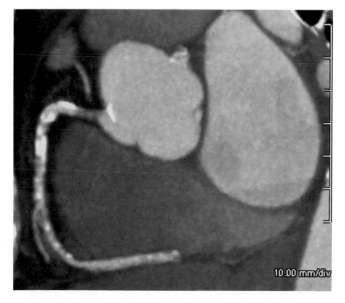

FIGURE C5.3 CT angiogram, anterior view of the right coronary artery: calcification is observed throughout the course of the vessel.

FIGURE C5.4 Stress (*top*) and rest (*bottom*) myocardial perfusion imaging study, vertical long-axis view. This demonstrates a fixed apical defect with subtle reversibility.

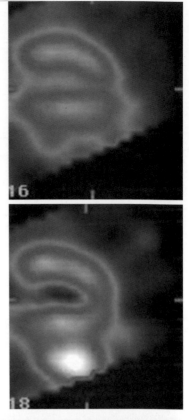

FIGURE C5.5 Stress (*top*) and rest (*bottom*) myocardial perfusion image, short axis view.

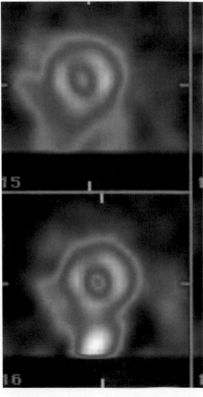

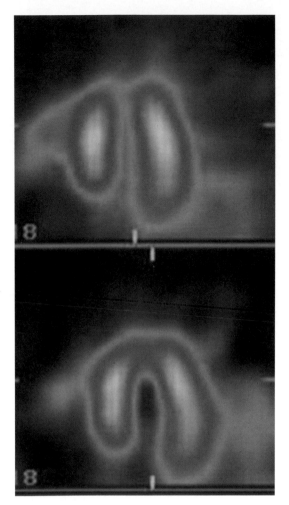

FIGURE C5.6   Stress (*top*) and rest (*bottom*) myocardial perfusion image, horizontal long-axis view.

CASE 6

Correlation Between Stress Test and Cardiac Catheterization

A 53-year-old woman, an avid runner, presents for self-referred CT angiography for "screening" for coronary artery disease. She denies cardiac symptoms at the time of the scan. On CT angiography, a complex atherosclerotic plaque is visualized in the proximal LAD, resulting in a luminal stenosis of 60%–70% (**Figure C6.1–C6.3**). The patient is referred to a cardiologist.

A detailed history reveals mild "chest pressure" while running, never occurring at rest. A stress myocardial perfusion study is ordered, which reveals a moderate sized reversible defect in the anterior wall (**Figure C6.4–C6.6**).

Subsequent cardiac catheterization reveals 80% stenoses in the proximal and mid LAD and the ostial diagonal branch (**Figure C6.7 and C6.8**). Percutaneous intervention is performed with two drug-eluting stents in the LAD and balloon angioplasty of the second diagonal branch.

On follow-up, the patient reports resolution of symptoms and increased exercise tolerance.

FIGURE C6.1   CT angiogram, anterior view. This displays the mixed plaque and severe disease in the LAD. LAD, left anterior descending artery.

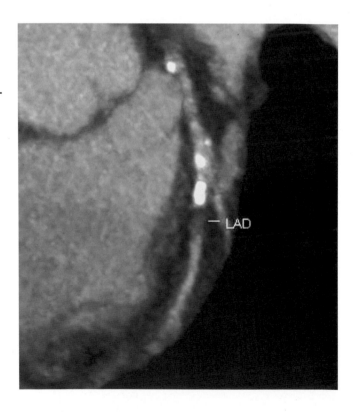

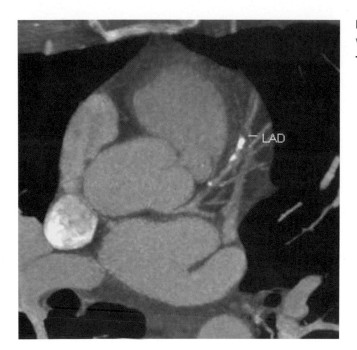

FIGURE C6.2   CT angiogram, foot (axial) view. LAD, left anterior descending artery.

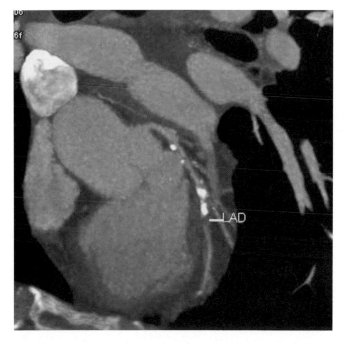

FIGURE C6.3   CT angiogram, right anterior oblique cranial view. LAD, left anterior descending artery.

FIGURE C6.4 Stress (*top*) and rest (*bottom*) myocardial perfusion imaging study, horizontal long axis view.

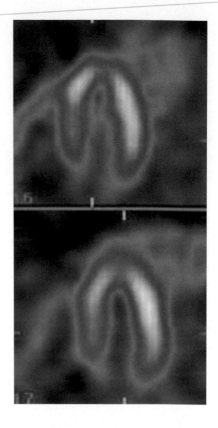

FIGURE C6.5 Stress (*top*) and rest (*bottom*) myocardial perfusion imaging study, short axis view.

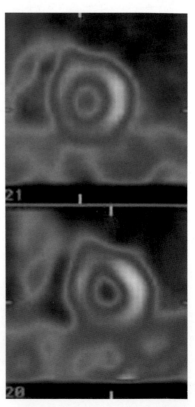

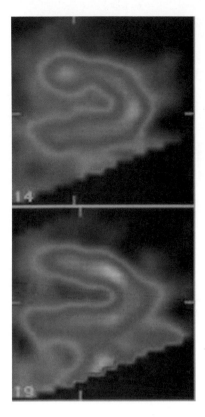

FIGURE C6.6   Stress (*top*) and rest (*bottom*) myocardial perfusion imaging study, vertical long axis view.

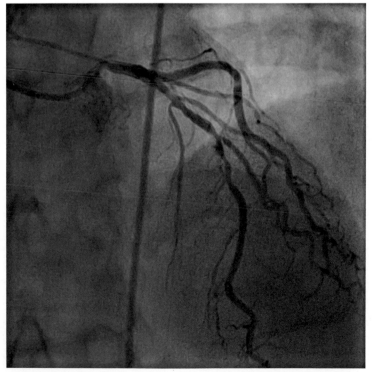

FIGURE C6.7   Coronary angiography, right anterior oblique caudal view.

FIGURE C6.8 Coronary angiography, right anterior oblique cranial view.

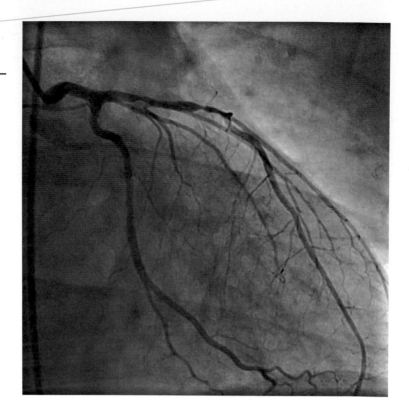

CASE 7

Atypical Symptoms With CTA Being the Definitive Diagnostic Test

An obese 61-year-old woman with a history of hyperlipidemia presents with "indigestion" symptoms for 6 months. She also reports progressive dyspnea on exertion for the same period of time. She undergoes a stress myocardial perfusion imaging study. During peak exercise, she has diagnostic ST-segment depression. However, perfusion images reveal no defect. She is referred for CT angiography.

On CTA, there is moderate to severe atherosclerotic disease in the ostial and proximal LAD (**Figure C7.1– C7.4**). For further evaluation and possible intervention for relief of symptoms, she is referred for cardiac catheterization.

Cardiac catheterization reveals 70% stenosis of the proximal LAD (**Figure C7.5**). Percutaneous intervention is performed with placement of a drug-eluting stent.

On follow-up, the dyspnea has improved tremendously with improvement in exercise tolerance. She continues to experience dyspepsia and responds to a trial of proton pump inhibitor therapy.

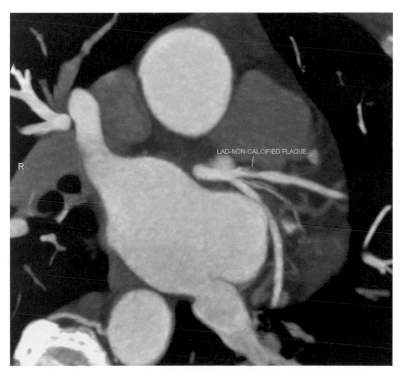

FIGURE C7.1   CT angiogram, left anterior oblique caudal view (axial). This displays the mixed atherosclerotic plaque in the proximal LAD. LAD, left anterior descending artery.

FIGURE C7.2 Coronary angiography, left anterior oblique caudal view.

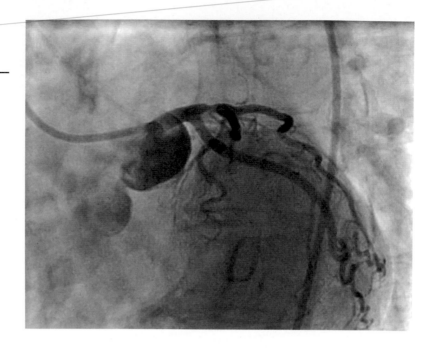

FIGURE C7.3 CT angiogram, right anterior oblique caudal view. LAD, left anterior descending artery.

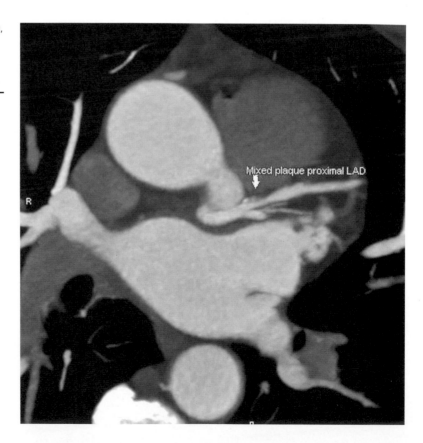

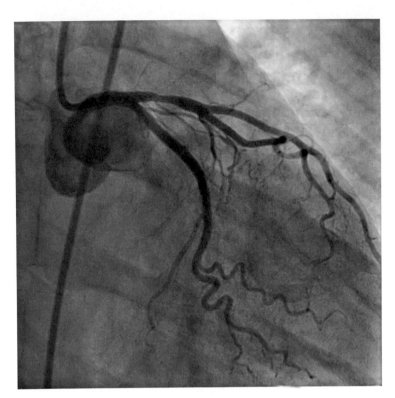

FIGURE C7.4 Coronary angiography, right anterior oblique caudal view.

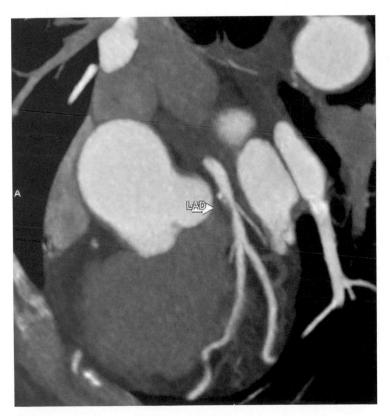

FIGURE C7.5 CT angiogram, left anterior oblique cranial view (anterior). The proximal, mid and distal segments of the LAD are visualized well. LAD, left anterior descending artery.

Diagnosis of CAD in a Patient Presenting to Emergency Center With Acute Chest Pain

A 52-year-old male with obesity and a history of ankylosing spondylitis has left arm numbness and chest discomfort with exertion for a few weeks. Finally, he presents to the emergency center for further evaluation. He undergoes a CTA.

CTA reveals a mixed atherosclerotic plaque consisting of calcified and non-calcified elements with a severity of greater than 70% in the proximal LAD (**Figure C8.1**). A serial lesion in the mid-LAD consists of a non-calcified plaque with severity greater than 70% (**Figure C8.2 and C8.3**). He is taken to the catheterization laboratory on an urgent basis.

Coronary angiography on cardiac catheterization reveals 80% stenosis of the mid LAD (**Figure C8.4–C8.6**). The small second diagonal branch is found to be occluded. Percutaneous intervention is performed and a drug-eluting stent is placed in the mid LAD. Aggressive medical therapy is commenced. He is discharged from the hospital in stable condition.

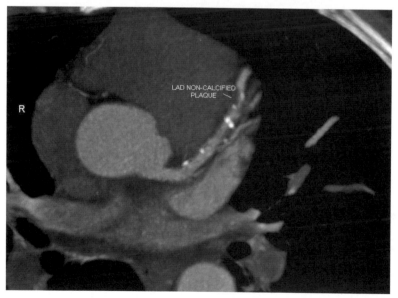

FIGURE C8.1 CT angiogram, left anterior oblique caudal view. This view displays the proximal and mid segments of the LAD. Focal areas of calcification are noted through its course. The proximal segment is visualized with the mixed atherosclerotic plaque. LAD, left anterior descending artery.

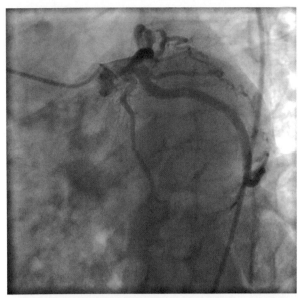

FIGURE C8.2 Coronary angiogram of the left coronary system, left anterior oblique caudal view.

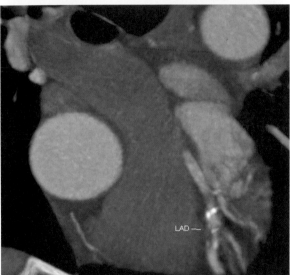

FIGURE C8.3 CT angiogram, left anterior oblique cranial view. This view displays the LAD in the traditional angiographic view. LAD, left anterior descending artery.

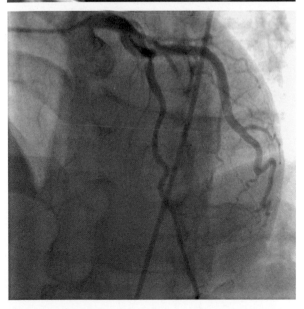

FIGURE C8.4 Coronary angiogram of the left coronary system, left anterior oblique cranial view.

FIGURE C8.5 CT angiogram, right anterior oblique cranial view. LAD, left anterior descending artery.

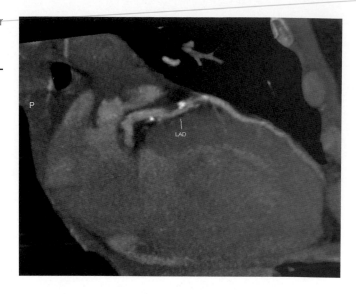

FIGURE C8.6 Coronary angiogram, right anterior oblique cranial view.

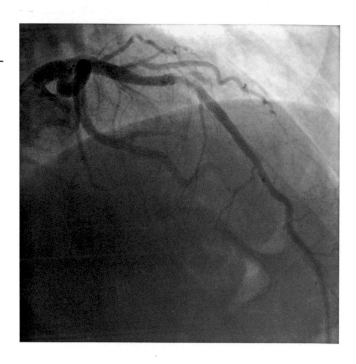

CASE 9

Diagnosis of Coronary Aneurysm and Correlation With Magnetic Resonance Imaging, Catheterization, and Pathology

A 61-year-old male with a history of coronary artery disease presents with recurrent chest pain. Five years prior to the index presentation, he underwent a cardiac catheterization for intractable chest pain and was found to have multiple small aneurysms of all three coronary arteries. The proximal circumflex artery was found to have significant disease and successful percutaneous intervention and stenting was performed.

After initial relief of symptoms, the patient presents with progressive chest pain. Cardiac catheterization is performed for further evaluation of progression of native disease and status of previous stent.

The stent in the circumflex artery is patent. The mid and distal segments of the circumflex reveal large saccular aneurysms (**Cine C9.1 and C9.2**). The RCA is found to contain a large fusiform aneurysm nearly 20 mm in diameter (**Cine C9.3**). The distal vessel is unable to fill. For evaluation of the aneurysm, a CTA is ordered.

CTA reveal large aneurysms of the mid and distal left circumflex artery, 10 mm and 12 mm in diameter, respectively (**Figure C9.1 and C9.2**). The RCA contains a large aneurysm, nearly 60 mm in diameter, containing a large, eccentric thrombus consistent with a dissection or contained rupture (**Figure C9.3**). There is also a severe atherosclerotic lesion observed distal to the aneurysm, greater than 70% in severity. After consultation with cardiothoracic surgeons, the patient consents to undergo coronary artery bypass grafting. A cardiac magnetic resonance image (MRI) is performed prior to surgery for evaluation of myocardial viability.

Cardiac MRI reveals a small area of infarction in the inferior wall with preserved left ventricular function. Images obtained by various weightings and contrast administration characterize the thrombus within the RCA aneurysm well (**Figure C9.4 and C9.5** and **Cine C9.5**). The thrombotic area measures nearly 5 cm at the widest dimension, occupying a large area of the aneurysm (nearly 6 cm at the widest diameter).

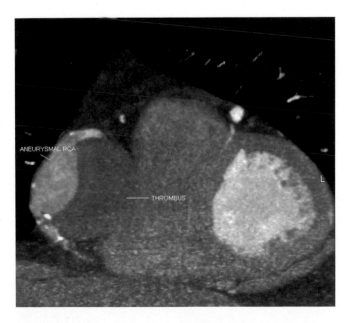

FIGURE C9.1 CT angiogram of the RCA, anterior view. The aneurysm is visualized well, surrounded by a large thrombotic area. RCA, right coronary artery.

FIGURE C9.2   CT angiogram of the left coronary system, right anterior oblique caudal view. The patent stent in the left circumflex artery as well as the ectatic changes are appreciated. LCX, left circumflex artery.

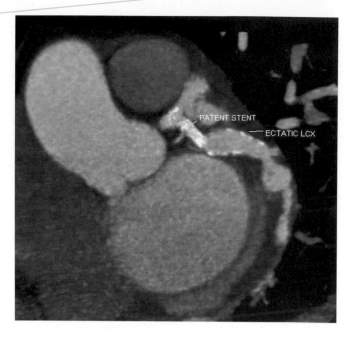

Successful bypass grafting and resection of the aneurysm is performed. Pathology confirms the mural thrombus, extensive fibrosis, and chronic inflammation in the wall of the aneurysm (**Figure C9.6 and C9.7**). The muscular artery specimen reveals myxoid degenerative changes. The patient is discharged in stable condition on postoperative day 8.

Video Clips: C9.1 Cineangiography of the left system, right anterior oblique caudal view. This demonstrates diffuse ectatic changes; **C9.2** Cineangiography of the left system, left anterior oblique caudal view; **C9.3** Cineangiography of the right coronary artery, right anterior oblique caudal view. Note the large aneurysm and inability to fill the distal vessel. "Swirling" of the contrast is noted; **C9.4** Cineangiography of the right coronary artery, left anterior oblique caudal view; **C9.5** First-pass perfusion cardiac magnetic resonance image. This demonstrates lack of uptake within the thrombotic area surrounding the right coronary artery aneurysm. ▣

FIGURE C9.3   CT angiogram of the LAD, right anterior oblique cranial view. LAD, left anterior descending artery.

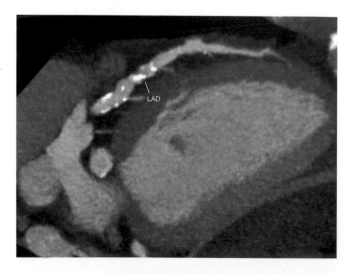

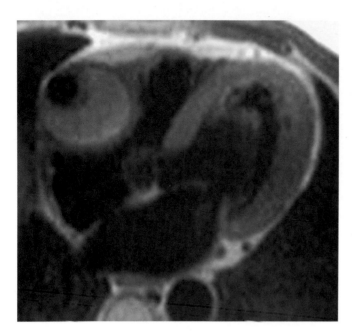

FIGURE C9.4 Cardiac magnetic resonance image, dark blood half-Fourier acquisition single-shot turbo spin-echo (HASTE) sequence. This demonstrates the thrombotic area as a higher signal intensity structure surrounding the blood pool within the aneurysm.

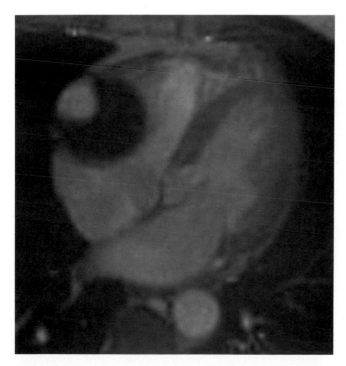

FIGURE C9.5 Cardiac magnetic resonance image, delayed hyperenhancement sequence. This image displays the thrombotic aneurysm as a structure of low signal intensity (dark) surrounding a lighter blood pool.

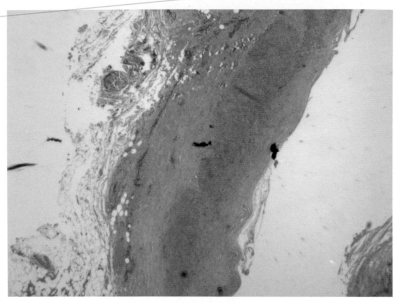

FIGURE C9.6   Coronary wall shows myxoid degeneration, calcification, fibrosis, and adventitial chronic inflammation (hematoxylin & eosin, original magnification ×125).
Image courtesy of Dr. Sharath Bhagavathi, MD, Department of Pathology, William Beaumont Hospital, Royal Oak, Michigan, USA.

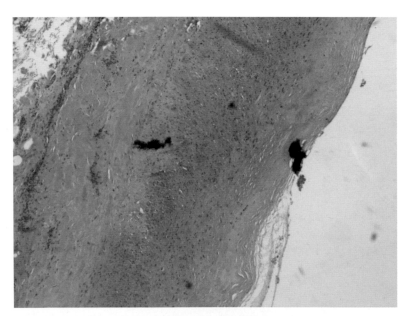

FIGURE C9.7   Higher magnification showing thrombus, myxoid degeneration, calcification, and chronic inflammation (hematoxylin & eosin, original magnification ×250).
Image courtesy of Dr. Sharath Bhagavathi, MD, Department of Pathology, William Beaumont Hospital, Royal Oak, Michigan, USA.

CASE 10

Limitation of Overlying Calcification—Correlation with Intravascular Ultrasound

A 63-year-old male with known coronary artery disease is referred for CTA. Fourteen years prior to the index visit, he sustained an anterior myocardial infarction and underwent four-vessel coronary artery bypass grafting surgery. For progressive symptoms of atypical chest discomfort, a CTA was ordered.

On CTA, all four grafts are found to be patent. However, the saphenous vein graft to the right coronary artery demonstrates a severe (80%) lesion in the proximal segment (**Figure C10.1 and C10.2**).

Subsequent coronary angiography confirms the findings (**Cine C10.1 and C10.2**). Percutaneous intervention and successful stenting of the lesion is performed (**Cine C10.3**).

Video Clips: C10.1 Cineangiography of the saphenous vein graft to the right coronary artery, left anterior oblique cranial view; **C10.2** Cineangiography of the saphenous vein graft to the right coronary artery, left anterior oblique caudal view; **C10.3** Cineangiography of the saphenous vein graft to right coronary artery, post-intervention.

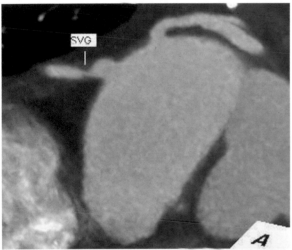

FIGURE C10.1   CT angiogram, left anterior oblique view. This demonstrates the severe lesion in the saphenous vein graft. SVG, saphenous vein graft.

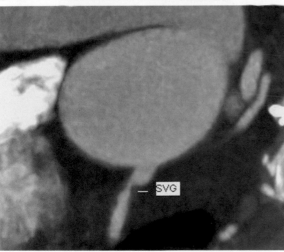

FIGURE C10.2   CT angiogram, right anterior oblique view. SVG, saphenous vein graft.

Bicuspid Aortic Valve

A 54-year-old African American male presents to the hospital with a 2-day history of left-sided chest pain. He has a history of nonischemic cardiomyopathy, hypertension, and a bicuspid aortic valve. The chest pain radiates to the left upper extremity and neck. The discomfort occurs at rest and is associated with shortness of breath. He is admitted to the hospital to rule out an acute coronary syndrome. No ECG changes are seen and cardiac enzymes are negative. He undergoes CT angiography to assess for significant coronary artery disease as a cause of his symptoms. CTA reveals a calcium score of 0 Agatston units, normal coronary arteries, bicuspid aortic valve, interatrial septal aneurysm, and moderate left ventricular dysfunction (**Cine C11.1 and C11.2**). Transthoracic echocardiogram also reveals a bicuspid aortic valve (**Cine C11.3 and C11.4**). He is discharged home after review of the CT angiograms.

Video Clips: C11.1 CT angiogram of a bicuspid aortic valve. There is calcification and fusion of the right and left coronary leaflets; **C11.2** Echocardiogram with similar short axis view of the aortic valve; **C11.3** CT angiogram demonstrating calcification and reduced mobility of one of the aortic valve leaflets and prolapse of the other leaflet; **C11.4** Echocardiogram with similar parasternal long axis view of the aortic valve.

CASE 12

Saphenous Vein Graft Pseudoaneurysm

A 71-year-old male presents to the hospital with shortness of breath of 3 weeks' duration. He has a history of coronary artery disease and two previous coronary bypass-grafting surgeries. He experiences the shortness of breath predominately while lying flat in bed and it is accompanied with chest tightness. Chest X-ray shows a questionable left perihilar mass. A 2D echocardiogram shows preserved left ventricular function, dilated aortic root, and a mass compressing the pulmonary artery. CT angiogram is preformed to better delineate the mass.

CT angiogram reveals severe native coronary artery disease and only one patent saphenous vein bypass graft, which has severe proximal disease and severe dilation distally. Because the vein graft came off the aorta, there is a large non-enhancing mass circumferential to the vein graft (**Figure C12.1**). In some views the mass appears to compress the pulmonary artery. Cardiac catheterization reveals an aneurysmal saphenous vein graft with significant disease (**Figure C12.2** and **Cine C12.1**). Intraoperative findings include a large pseudoaneurysm of the saphenous vein graft with thrombus-like material within it. The patient undergoes redo–coronary artery bypass graft (CABG) along with aneurysmectomy of the saphenous vein graft pseudoaneurysm. He is unable to be weaned from the bypass pump and expires in the operating room.

Video Clip: C12.1 Cineangiogram of the aneurysmal saphenous vein graft.

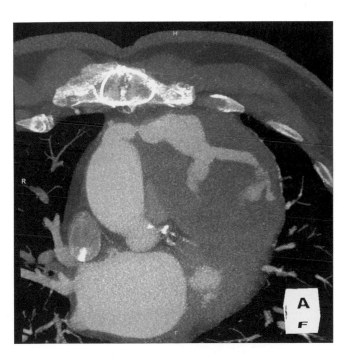

FIGURE C12.1 CT angiogram demonstrates an aneursymal saphenous vein graft with a large circumferential non-enhancing mass.

FIGURE C12.2 Cineangiogram of the aneurysmal saphenous vein graft.

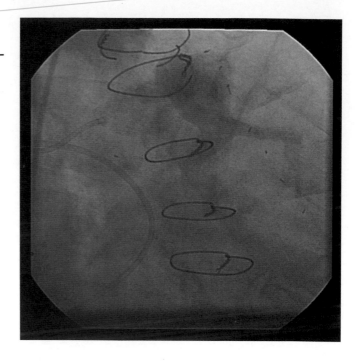

CASE 13

Occluded Right Coronary Artery With an Aneurysm of the Mid Inferior Wall

A 64-year-old male with a history of hyperlipidemia and significant tobacco abuse, who has been experiencing chest burning that he attributed to gastroesophageal reflux, is admitted to the chest pain unit for further diagnostic workup. He undergoes an exercise MPI study that demonstrates an inferior wall infarct. Subsequently, he is referred for a CT angiogram.

The CT angiogram demonstrates a significantly elevated calcium score of 1329 Agatston units. Heavy calcified plaque involves the proximal left anterior descending artery and results in approximately 70% luminal narrowing (**Figure C13.1**). The left circumflex artery has focal areas of calcification extending into the first and second obtuse marginal vessels. There is a severe complex atherosclerotic plaque (calcified and non-calcified) extending from the ostium of the right coronary artery to the mid segment. The right coronary is occluded in the mid segment, and the distal segment is filled via collateral vessels (**Figure C13.2**). In addition, the gated cine images reveal an inferior wall myocardial infarction with an associated aneurysm (**Figures C13.3 and C13.4** and **Cine C13.1**). The patient is medically treated and discharged home. He will undergo coronary artery bypass grafting at a later date.

Video Clip C13.1 CT angiogram (right anterior oblique view) demonstrating an aneurysm of the mid inferior wall.

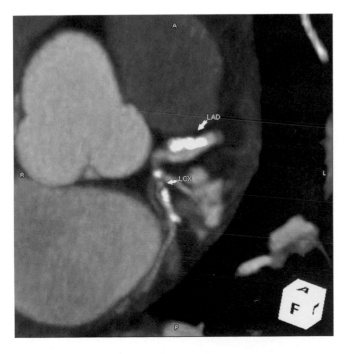

FIGURE C13.1 CT angiogram (left anterior oblique view) reveals heavy calcification within the proximal left anterior descending and proximal left circumflex arteries. LAD, left anterior descending artery; LCX, left circumflex artery.

FIGURE C13.2 CT angiogram (left anterior oblique view) demonstrates heavy calcification in the proximal right coronary artery and an occluded mid right coronary artery.

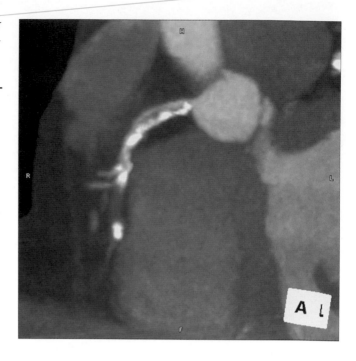

FIGURE C13.3 CT angiogram (right anterior oblique view) demonstrating an aneurysm of the mid inferior wall during diastole.

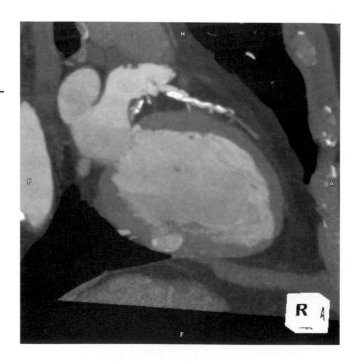

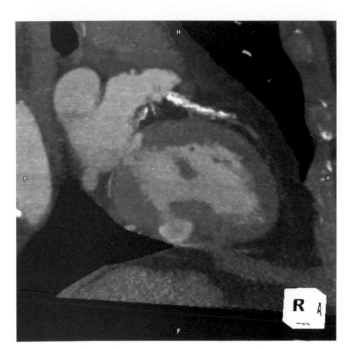

FIGURE C13.4 CT angiogram (right anterior oblique view) demonstrating an aneurysm of the mid inferior wall during systole.

CASE 14

Image Reconstruction Artifact of the Right Coronary Artery

A 61-year-old female who has a prior history of cerebrovascular accident, gastroesophageal reflux disease, and nonsustained ventricular tachycardia presents to the hospital with intermittent substernal chest pain, dyspnea, diaphoresis, and lightheadedness. She undergoes CT angiography and is initially felt to have a severe (80% luminal stenosis) non-calcified eccentric plaque within the proximal right coronary artery (**Figure C14.1**). The remaining segments of the coronary tree are normal. She undergoes cardiac catheterization, which reveals preserved left ventricular function with normal coronary arteries, including the proximal right coronary artery (**Figure C14.2** and **Cine C14.1**). Reanalysis of the CT angiograms reveals significant disease in the proximal right coronary artery on the 75% reconstruction interval images (**Figure C14.1**) and no disease in the same segment on the 65% reconstruction interval images (**Figure C14.3**).

Video Clip C14.1 Cardiac catheterization demonstrating a normal right coronary artery.

FIGURE C14.1 CT angiogram, 75% reconstruction interval image. Left anterior oblique cranial view demonstrating significant disease within the proximal right coronary artery. RCA, right coronary artery.

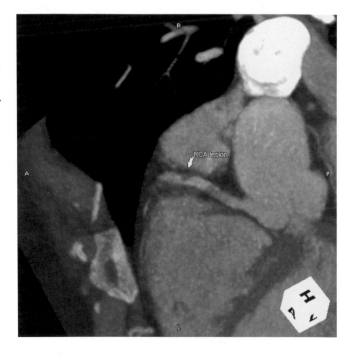

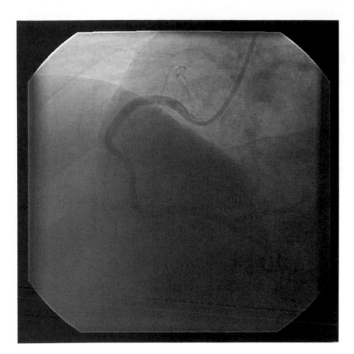

FIGURE C14.2 Cardiac catheterization demonstrating a normal right coronary artery.

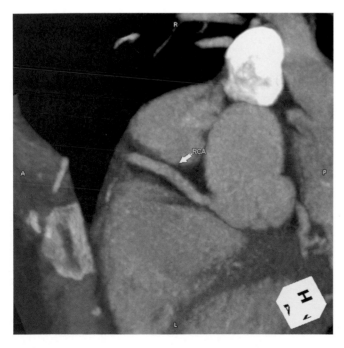

FIGURE C14.3 CT angiogram, 65% reconstruction interval image. Left anterior oblique cranial view demonstrating no disease within the proximal right coronary artery. RCA, right coronary artery.

CASE 15

Focal Stenosis of the Circumflex Artery With Cardiac Catheterization Correlation

A 41-year-old male with a history of hypertension, hypercholesterolemia, and tobacco abuse presents to the hospital with chest pain radiating to the left shoulder of 5 days' duration. Stress MPI demonstrates his ability to exercise 9.5 minutes on the Bruce protocol without any ECG changes, symptoms, or perfusion abnormalities. He is discharged home. He follows up with his cardiologist and is scheduled for a CT angiography because of ongoing symptoms.

CT angiography reveals a calcium score of 16.2 Agatston units, anomalous origin of the right coronary artery, and significant concentric non-calcified plaque (90% stenosis) in the left circumflex artery (**Figures C15.1 and C15.2**). Cardiac catheterization reveals similar findings (**Figures C15.3 and C15.4** and **Cine C15.1 and C15.2**). The lesion in the left circumflex artery is successfully treated with a drug-eluting stent and the stenosis is reduced from 95% to 0%. The patient's symptoms abate following the procedure.

Video Clips: C15.1 Cineangiogram in the caudal view demonstrates significant disease within the left circumflex artery; **C15.2** Cineangiogram in the left anterior oblique view demonstrates significant disease within the left circumflex artery.

FIGURE C15.1   CT angiography in the caudal view demonstrates significant concentric non-calcified plaque within the left circumflex artery. LCX, left circumflex artery.

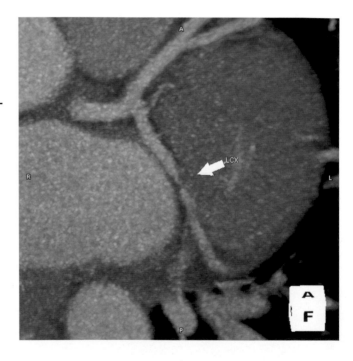

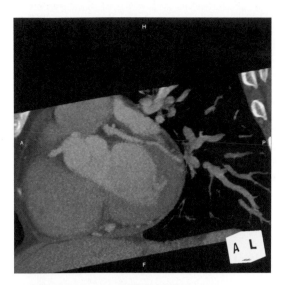

FIGURE C15.2   CT angiography in the left anterior oblique view demonstrates significant concentric non-calcified plaque within the left circumflex artery.

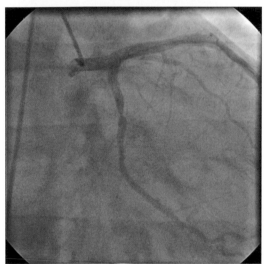

FIGURE C15.3   Cineangiogram in the caudal view demonstrates significant disease within the left circumflex artery.

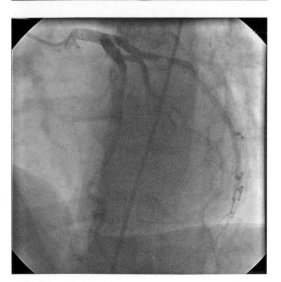

FIGURE C15.4   Cineangiogram in the left anterior oblique view demonstrates significant disease within the circumflex artery.

Blooming Artifact in Focally Calicified Segments

A 52-year-old female with a history of hypertension and hypothyroidism presents to the office with complaints of atypical chest discomfort. She has a long-standing history of noncardiac chest pain and underwent a normal stress echocardiogram 9 months previous to this office visit. She is scheduled to undergo a CT angiogram to definitively exclude coronary atherosclerosis as a cause of her symptoms.

CT angiography reveals a calcium score of 326 Agatston units, with moderate calcification within the distal left main coronary artery and significant calcification in the proximal left anterior descending artery (**Figure C16.1**). She undergoes an exercise MPI and is found to have no evidence of ischemia. Because of ongoing symptoms and the possibility of balanced ischemia on the MPI, she is scheduled for a cardiac catheterization. Cardiac catheterization reveals no significant disease within the distal left main coronary artery and left anterior descending artery (**Figure C16.2** and **Cine C16.1**).

Video Clip: C16.1 Cardiac catheterization in the right anterior oblique caudal view reveals no significant disease within the distal left main coronary artery and left anterior descending artery.

FIGURE C16.1 CT angiogram in the right anterior oblique caudal view showing significant calcification within the distal left main coronary artery and left anterior descending artery. LAD, left anterior descending artery; LCX, left circumflex artery.

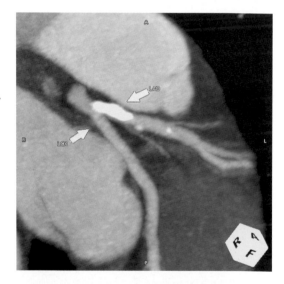

FIGURE C16.2 Cardiac catheterization in the right anterior oblique caudal view reveals no significant disease within the distal left main coronary artery and left anterior descending artery.

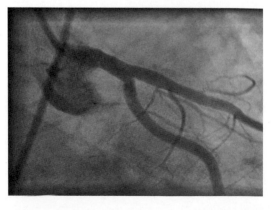

CASE 17

Correlation of a Subtotal Occlusion on CTA With Cardiac Catheterization

A 43-year-old male with a significant history of smoking presents to the hospital with stuttering chest pain of several days' duration. The chest pain starts in his anterior chest and radiates to the neck. Each episode of chest pain lasts 5–10 minutes. In the emergency room, serial enzymes and ECGs are not suggestive of an acute myocardial infarction, so he is scheduled for an urgent CT angiogram.

The CT angiogram demonstrates a calcium score of 0 Agatston units, normal left coronary system, and occlusion of the proximal to mid right coronary artery with faint opacification of the distal right coronary artery (**Figure C17.1**). He is admitted to the hospital and undergoes cardiac catheterization the next day. Cineangiogram reveals a normal left coronary system with a focal subtotal occlusion of the proximal right coronary artery (**Figure C17.2** and **Cine C17.1**). He undergoes successful angioplasty and drug-eluting stenting of the right coronary artery, reducing the stenosis from 99% to 0% (**Figure C17.3** and **Cine C17.2**).

Video Clips: C17.1 Cineangiogram reveals a subtotal occlusion of the proximal/mid right coronary artery; **C17.2** Cineangiogram reveals a patent stent.

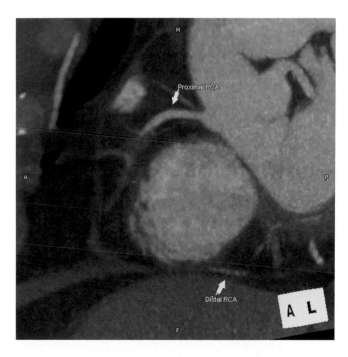

FIGURE C17.1   CT angiogram of the right coronary artery in the left anterior oblique view. The proximal/mid right coronary artery appears to be occluded without evidence of calcification. Just distal to the lesion, the mid right coronary artery is opacified and the distal right coronary artery is opacified. RCA, right coronary artery.

FIGURE C17.2 Cineangiogram reveals a subtotal occlusion of the proximal/mid right coronary artery.

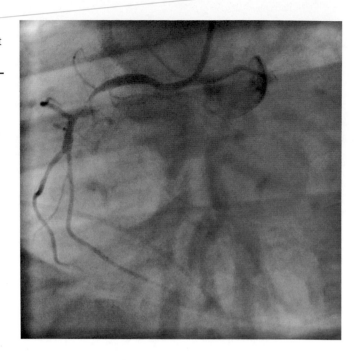

FIGURE C17.3 Cineangiogram reveals a patent stent.

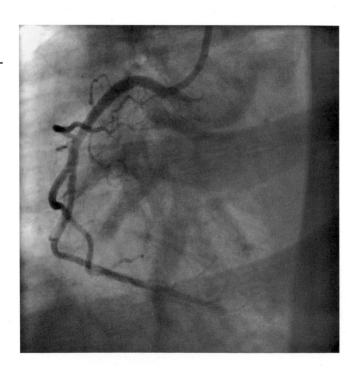

Occluded Stent With Collaterals

A 57-year-old man with coronary artery disease and prior percutaneous coronary intervention presents with atypical chest pain. Two years prior to presentation, he had sustained an inferior myocardial infarction treated with primary angioplasty. A CTA is ordered to evaluate for progression of native disease and stent patency.

On CTA, severe disease in the RCA is appreciated proximal to the stent (**Figures C18.1 and C18.2**). Reconstruction of images is performed at a higher (sharper) kernel (B46). With adequate (wide) windowing, occlusion of the stent is well-appreciated (**Figure C18.3**). The distal RCA fills via collaterals from the left circumflex artery (arrow, **Figure C18.4, Cine C18.1 and Cine C18.2**).

Medical therapy is instituted. The patient does well.

Video Clips: C18.1 Cineangiography of the left coronary system. Collaterals to the right are seen; **C18.2** Cineangiography of the right coronary artery demonstrating the occluded stent and distal filling via collaterals.

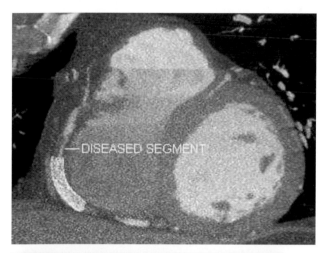

FIGURE C18.1 CT angiogram of the right coronary artery. No contrast is visualized within the stent.

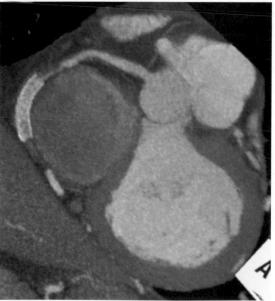

FIGURE C18.2 CT angiogram of the right coronary artery, left anterior oblique caudal view.

FIGURE C18.3 CT angiogram of the RCA, axial view. This image is reconstructed at a higher kernel and viewed with wide windowing. The struts of the stent are visualized well, with lack of contrast within. RCA, right coronary artery.

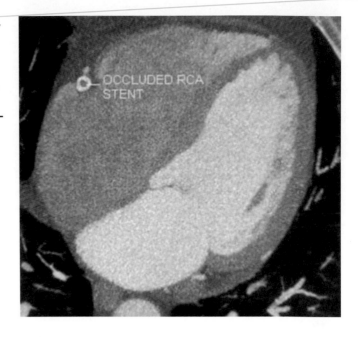

FIGURE C18.4 CT angiogram of the distal right coronary artery, axial view. The posterior descending artery is seen well, with retrograde filling presumably via collaterals.

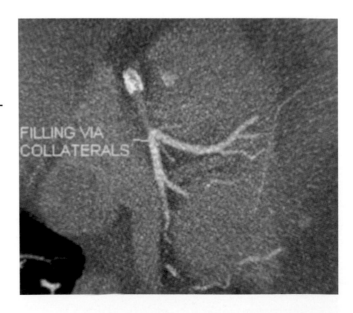

CASE 19

Severe CAD With IVUS Correlation

A 53-year-old woman with multiple coronary risk factors presents with atypical angina. A stress/rest myocardial perfusion imaging study is inconclusive. She is referred for a CTA.

On CTA, the mid segment of the LAD is found to be diffusely diseased. The stenosis in this area is difficult to assess because of overlying calcification. It is interpreted as moderate to severe disease (**Figures C19.1 and C19.2**).

On subsequent coronary angiography, there is mild to moderate disease in the mid-LAD (**Cine C19.1 and C19.2**). Intravascular ultrasound is performed, revealing severe (80%) disease in this segment (**Cine C19.3**). Percutaneous intervention is successfully performed and aggressive medical therapy for risk-factor modification is instituted. The patient's atypical symptoms resolve.

Video Clips: C19.1 Cineangiography of the left coronary system, right anterior oblique caudal view; **C19.2** Cineangiography of the left coronary system, right anterior oblique cranial view; **C19.3** Intravascular ultrasound of the mid and proximal left anterior descending artery.

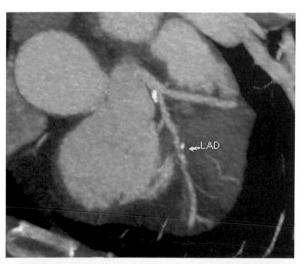

FIGURE C19.1   CT angiogram, right anterior oblique view. This displays the proximal and mid segments of the LAD with severe disease in the mid segment. LAD, left anterior descending artery.

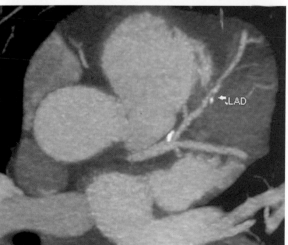

FIGURE C19.2   CT angiogram, axial view. LAD, left anterior descending artery.

5.3 Clinical Indications and Limitations

Kusai S. Aziz

The use of cardiac CT has significantly increased during the last few years because of advanced technology and the introduction of new generation 64-slice CT scans that enable higher spatial resolution and less motion artifact. Cardiac software has also advanced and made it much easier to calculate calcium scores and track coronary arteries and evaluate them in multiple orientations.

In 2006, the ACCF/ACR/SCCT/SCMR/ASNC/NASCI/SCAI/SIR published appropriateness criteria for both cardiac CT and cardiac MRI (Table 1–Table 7).[1] We recommend following these criteria since they represent the most evidence-based analysis of the rapidly increasing applications of this technology. However, it should be kept in mind that reimbursement of these studies by third-party payers remains very restricted. It should also be kept in mind that, considering the radiation exposure, cardiac CTA can not be recommended as a screening tool in middle age asymptomatic subjects.[2]

Limitations

Despite technological advances and the introduction of the 64-slice CT, this technology still faces many challenges that continue to limit its use. Severe calcifications remain one of these challenges, as they preclude accurate evaluation of the degree of stenosis. The presence of stents can also be a limiting factor, although this is much less of an obstacle than it was with 16-slice CT. High dose radiation is another limitation that should be kept in mind, because the radiation dose to the patient tends to increase from 16- to 64-slice CT. Patient radiation exposure in ECG-gated acquisitions may reach up to 40 mSv,[3] which exceeds the amount of radiation received during cardiac catheterization and selective coronary angiography, as well as that of percutaneous coronary angioplasty followed by stent placement (9.0 mSv).[4] Finally, it should be kept in mind that this technique uses contrast that can put patients at risk of contrast-induced nephropathy. This subject is discussed in a different chapter.

TABLE 5.1	Detection of CAD: Symptomatic	
Indication		**Appropriateness Criteria (Median Score)**
Evaluation of Chest Pain Syndrome (Use of CT Angiogram)		
1.	• Intermediate pre-test probability of CAD • ECG interpretable AND able to exercise	**U (5)**
2.	• Intermediate pre-test probability of CAD • ECG uninterpretable OR unable to exercise	**A (7)**
3.	• High pre-test probability of CAD	**I (2)**
Evaluation of Intra-Cardiac Structures (Use of CT Angiogram)		
4.	• Evaluation of suspected coronary anomalies	**A (9)**
Acute Chest Pain (Use of CT Angiogram)		
5.	• Low pre-test probability of CAD • No ECG changes and serial enzymes negative	**U (5)**

(Continued)

TABLE 5.1   Detection of CAD: Symptomatic (*Continued*)

Indication		Appropriateness Criteria (Median Score)
Acute Chest Pain (Use of CT Angiogram) (*Continued*)		
6.	• Intermediate pre-test probability of CAD • No ECG changes and serial enzymes negative	A (7)
7.	• High pre-test probability of CAD • No ECG changes and serial enzymes negative	U (6)
8.	• High pre-test probability of CAD • ECG—ST-segment elevation and/or positive cardiac enzymes	I (1)
9.	• "Triple rule out"—exclude obstructive CAD, aortic dissection, and pulmonary embolism • Intermediate pre-test probability for one of the above • ECG—no ST-segment elevation and initial enzymes negative	U (4)

Reprinted from Hendel RC, Patel MR, Kramer CM, et al. ACCF/ACR/SCCT/SCMR/ASNC/NASCI/SCAI/SIR 2006 appropriateness criteria for cardiac computed tomography and cardiac magnetic resonance imaging: a report of the American College of Cardiology Foundation Quality Strategic Directions Committee Appropriateness Criteria Working Group, American College of Radiology, Society of Cardiovascular Computed Tomography, Society for Cardiovascular Magnetic Resonance, American Society of Nuclear Cardiology, North American Society for Cardiac Imaging, Society for Cardiovascular Angiography and Interventions, and Society of Interventional Radiology. *J Am Coll Cardiol* 2006;48:1475–97, with permission from Elsevier.

TABLE 5.2   Detection of CAD: Asymptomatic (Without Chest Pain Syndrome)

Indication		Appropriateness Criteria (Median Score)
Asymptomatic (Use of CT Angiogram)		
10.	• Low CHD risk (Framingham risk criteria)	I (1)
11.	• Moderate CHD risk (Framingham)	I (2)
12.	• High CHD risk (Framingham)	U (4)

Reprinted from Hendel RC, Patel MR, Kramer CM, et al. ACCF/ACR/SCCT/SCMR/ASNC/NASCI/SCAI/SIR 2006 appropriateness criteria for cardiac computed tomography and cardiac magnetic resonance imaging: a report of the American College of Cardiology Foundation Quality Strategic Directions Committee Appropriateness Criteria Working Group, American College of Radiology, Society of Cardiovascular Computed Tomography, Society for Cardiovascular Magnetic Resonance, American Society of Nuclear Cardiology, North American Society for Cardiac Imaging, Society for Cardiovascular Angiography and Interventions, and Society of Interventional Radiology. *J Am Coll Cardiol* 2006;48:1475–97, with permission from Elsevier.

TABLE 5.3   Risk Assessment: General Population

Indication		Appropriateness Criteria (Median Score)
Asymptomatic (Calcium Scoring)		
13.	• Low CHD risk (Framingham)	I (1)
14.	• Moderate CHD risk (Framingham)	U (6)
15.	• High CHD risk (Framingham)	U (5)

Reprinted from Hendel RC, Patel MR, Kramer CM, et al. ACCF/ACR/SCCT/SCMR/ASNC/NASCI/SCAI/SIR 2006 appropriateness criteria for cardiac computed tomography and cardiac magnetic resonance imaging: a report of the American College of Cardiology Foundation Quality Strategic Directions Committee Appropriateness Criteria Working Group, American College of Radiology, Society of Cardiovascular Computed Tomography, Society for Cardiovascular Magnetic Resonance, American Society of Nuclear Cardiology, North American Society for Cardiac Imaging, Society for Cardiovascular Angiography and Interventions, and Society of Interventional Radiology. *J Am Coll Cardiol* 2006;48:1475–97, with permission from Elsevier.

TABLE 5.4	Detection of CAD With Prior Test Results	
Indication		Appropriateness Criteria (Median Score)
Evaluation of Chest Pain Syndrome (Use of CT Angiogram)		
16.	• Uninterpretable or equivocal stress test (exercise, perfusion, or stress echo)	**A (8)**
17.	• Evidence of moderate to severe ischemia on stress test (exercise, perfusion, or stress echo)	**I (2)**

Reprinted from Hendel RC, Patel MR, Kramer CM, et al. ACCF/ACR/SCCT/SCMR/ASNC/NASCI/SCAI/SIR 2006 appropriateness criteria for cardiac computed tomography and cardiac magnetic resonance imaging: a report of the American College of Cardiology Foundation Quality Strategic Directions Committee Appropriateness Criteria Working Group, American College of Radiology, Society of Cardiovascular Computed Tomography, Society for Cardiovascular Magnetic Resonance, American Society of Nuclear Cardiology, North American Society for Cardiac Imaging, Society for Cardiovascular Angiography and Interventions, and Society of Interventional Radiology. *J Am Coll Cardiol* 2006;48:1475–97, with permission from Elsevier.

TABLE 5.5	Risk Assessment With Prior Test Results	
Indication		Appropriateness Criteria (Median Score)
Asymptomatic (Calcium Scoring)		
18.	• Prior calcium score within previous 5 years	**I (1)**
Asymptomatic (Use of CT Angiogram)		
19.	• High CHD risk (Framingham) • Within 2 years prior cardiac CT angiogram or invasive angiogram without significant obstructive disease	**I (2)**
20.	• High CHD risk (Framingham) • Prior calcium score greater than or equal to 400	**I (3)**

Reprinted from Hendel RC, Patel MR, Kramer CM, et al. ACCF/ACR/SCCT/SCMR/ASNC/NASCI/SCAI/SIR 2006 appropriateness criteria for cardiac computed tomography and cardiac magnetic resonance imaging: a report of the American College of Cardiology Foundation Quality Strategic Directions Committee Appropriateness Criteria Working Group, American College of Radiology, Society of Cardiovascular Computed Tomography, Society for Cardiovascular Magnetic Resonance, American Society of Nuclear Cardiology, North American Society for Cardiac Imaging, Society for Cardiovascular Angiography and Interventions, and Society of Interventional Radiology. *J Am Coll Cardiol* 2006;48:1475–97, with permission from Elsevier.

TABLE 5.6	Risk Assessment: Preoperative Evaluation for Non-Cardiac Surgery	
Indication		Appropriateness Criteria (Median Score)
Low-Risk Surgery (Use of CT Angiogram)		
21.	• Intermediate perioperative risk	**I (1)**
Intermediate- or High-Risk Surgery (Use of CT Angiogram)		
22.	• Intermediate perioperative risk	**U (4)**

Reprinted from Hendel RC, Patel MR, Kramer CM, et al. ACCF/ACR/SCCT/SCMR/ASNC/NASCI/SCAI/SIR 2006 appropriateness criteria for cardiac computed tomography and cardiac magnetic resonance imaging: a report of the American College of Cardiology Foundation Quality Strategic Directions Committee Appropriateness Criteria Working Group, American College of Radiology, Society of Cardiovascular Computed Tomography, Society for Cardiovascular Magnetic Resonance, American Society of Nuclear Cardiology, North American Society for Cardiac Imaging, Society for Cardiovascular Angiography and Interventions, and Society of Interventional Radiology. *J Am Coll Cardiol* 2006;48:1475–97, with permission from Elsevier.

TABLE 5.7	Detection of CAD: Post-Revascularization (PCI or CABG)	
Indication		**Appropriateness Criteria (Median Score)**
Evaluation of Chest Pain Syndrome (Use of CT Angiogram)		
23.	• Evaluation of bypass grafts and coronary anatomy	**U (6)**
24.	• History of percutaneous revascularization with stents	**U (5)**
Asymptomatic (Use of CT Angiogram)		
25.	• Evaluation of bypass grafts and coronary anatomy • Less than 5 years after CABG	**I (2)**
26.	• Evaluation of bypass grafts and coronary anatomy • Greater than or equal to 5 years after CABG	**I (3)**
27.	• Evaluation for in-stent restenosis and coronary anatomy after PCI	**I (2)**

Reprinted from Hendel RC, Patel MR, Kramer CM, et al. ACCF/ACR/SCCT/SCMR/ASNC/NASCI/SCAI/SIR 2006 appropriateness criteria for cardiac computed tomography and cardiac magnetic resonance imaging: a report of the American College of Cardiology Foundation Quality Strategic Directions Committee Appropriateness Criteria Working Group, American College of Radiology, Society of Cardiovascular Computed Tomography, Society for Cardiovascular Magnetic Resonance, American Society of Nuclear Cardiology, North American Society for Cardiac Imaging, Society for Cardiovascular Angiography and Interventions, and Society of Interventional Radiology. *J Am Coll Cardiol* 2006,48:1475–97, with permission from Elsevier.

REFERENCES

1. Hendel RC, Patel MR, Kramer CM, et al. ACCF/ACR/SCCT/SCMR/ASNC/NASCI/SCAI/SIR 2006 appropriateness criteria for cardiac computed tomography and cardiac magnetic resonance imaging: A report of the American College of Cardiology Foundation Quality Strategic Directions Committee Appropriateness Criteria Working Group, American College of Radiology, Society of Cardiovascular Computed Tomography, Society for Cardiovascular Magnetic Resonance, American Society of Nuclear Cardiology, North American Society for Cardiac Imaging, Society for Cardiovascular Angiography and Interventions, and Society of Interventional Radiology. *J Am Coll Cardiol.* 2006; 48:1475–1497.
2. Choi EK, Choi SI, et al. Coronary computed tomography angiography as a screening tool for the detection of occult coronary artery disease in asymptomatic individuals. *J Am Coll Cardiol.* 2008; 52:357–365.
3. Paul JF, Abada H T. Strategies for reduction of radiation dose in cardiac multislice CT. *Eur Radiol.* 2007; 17:2028–2037.
4. Betsou S, Efstathopoulos EP, Katritsis D, Faulkner K, Panayiotakis G. Patient radiation doses during cardiac catheterization procedures. *Br J Radiol.* 1998; 71:634–639.

5.4 Iodinated Radiocontrast Agents

Ibrahim Shah, Kevin L. Berger, and George S. Abela

Radiocontrast agents are compounds used to improve the visibility of internal bodily structures in an X-ray image. Iodine, because of its high atomic number, effectively absorbs X-rays and appears radio-opaque in an X-ray image. Since iodine-based contrasts are used in computed tomography angiography (CTA), the focus of this chapter is iodine-based contrast media.

TABLE 5.8	Classification of Contrast Media					
	Generic Name	**Benzene Ring**	**Iodine to Particle Ratio**	**Osmolality (mOsm/kg)**	**Viscosity at 37°C**	
Ionic	Diatrizoate (Hypaque, Renografin, Angiovist)	Monomer	1.5	1800–2100	8.4	**High Osmolar**
	Ioxaglate (Hexabrix)	Dimer	3	600	7.5	
Nonionic	Iohexol (Omnipaque)	Monomer	3	700–840	8–10.5	**Low Osmolar**
	Iopamidol (Isovue)	Monomer	3			
	Ioversol (Optiray)	Monomer	3			
	Iodixanol (Visipaque)	Dimer	6	280	12	**Iso-osmolar**

Classification

In 1929 the first organic iodide preparation (Selectan) was explored, which contained one iodine atom per benzoic acid ring. All iodinated radiocontrast agents are derivatives of benzoic acid, but the number of iodine molecules, the ionic and osmolar composition, and the viscosity vary among different agents. Iodinated contrast agents are divided into those that ionize in solution (ionic agents) and those that do not (nonionic agents) (Table 5.8).

For CTA, the usual amount of contrast agent used is about 100 mL and an iodine concentration of 320–370 mg/mL is required for left ventricular and coronary contrast injection. The higher the number of iodine molecules attached to a benzene ring, the lower the concentration of the solution needed to be an effective radiocontrast, and hence the lower the osmolality. These agents are divided into three categories on the basis of osmolality (Figure 5.11):

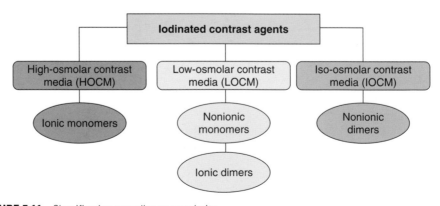

FIGURE 5.11 Classification according to osmolarity.

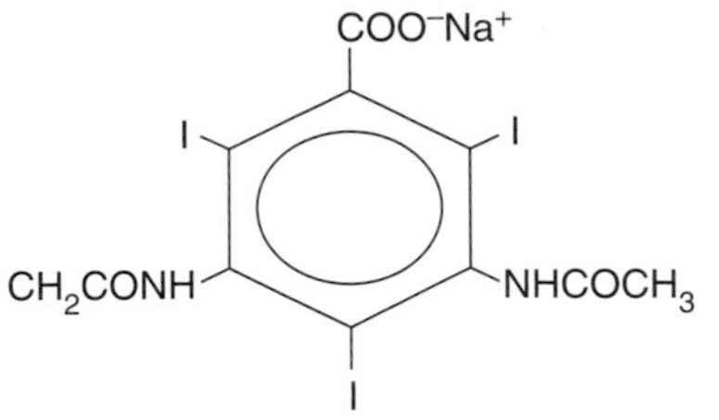

FIGURE 5.12   High-osmolar ionic agent, ratio 1.5 (3:2).

- High-osmolar contrast media (HOCM)
- Low-osmolar contrast media (LOCM)
- Iso-osmolar contrast media (IOCM)

High-Osmolar Contrast Media

These agents are monomeric salts of tri-iodinated benzoic acid. The iodine atoms are attached at position 2, 4, 6 of the benzene ring and position 1 has a cation, either sodium or methyl-glucamine (Figure 5.12).

These agents contain three iodine atoms for every two osmotically active ions, i.e., the substituted benzoic acid ring and the cation at position 1, and thus are considered ratio 1.5 agents. They are markedly hypertonic with an osmolality >1500 mOsm or approximately six times higher than plasma.

Renografin contains sodium citrate and sodium ethylenediaminetetraacetic acid (EDTA) as additives, which has calcium-binding properties. Angiovist, on the other hand, has calcium EDTA as its additive to overcome the calcium-binding effects.

The hypertonicity and calcium-chelating properties of these compounds contribute to their side effects.[1]

Low-Osmolar Contrast Media

These agents have three atoms of iodine for each ion. Being a ratio of 3:1, they are only two to three times the osmolality of plasma. Hence, they are referred to as low-osmolar contrast agents (LOCM). These agents are either nonionic monomers or ionic dimers. There is some evidence that LOCM produce fewer allergic side effects and are less nephrotoxic, but this has been difficult to confirm in large clinical studies.[2]

Ionic Dimers

An ionic dimer is created by the formation of a dimer in which six iodine atoms are associated with two osmotically active agents and hence are ratio 3 (Figure 5.13). The osmolality is

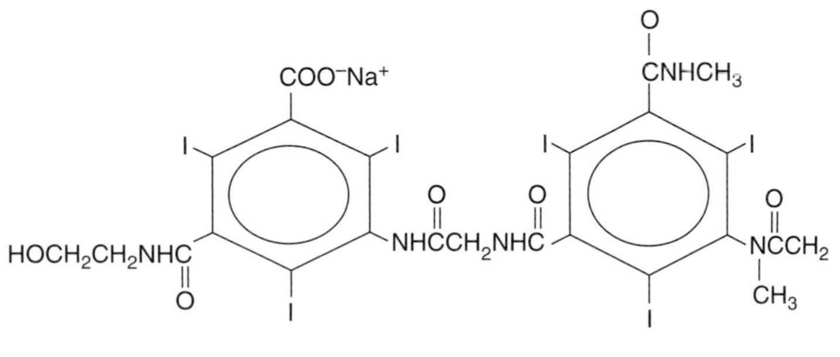

FIGURE 5.13   Low-osmolar ionic dimer, ratio 3 (6:2).

FIGURE 5.14 Low-osmolar nonionic monomer, ratio 3 (3:1).

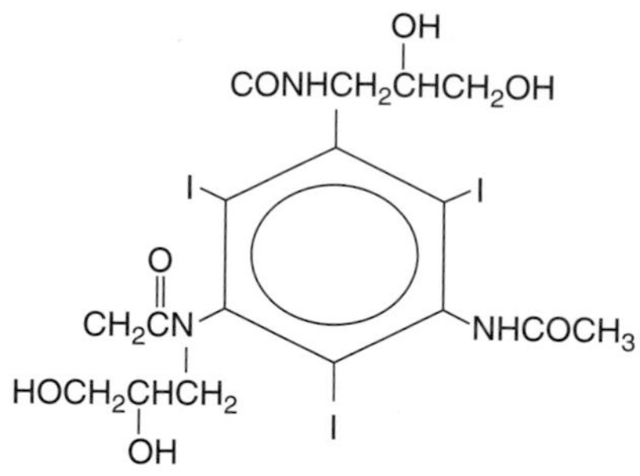

substantially reduced (~600 mOsm/kg). Because of the low osmolality of these agents, they have fewer side effects.[3] An example is ioxaglate (Hexabrix).

Nonionic Monomers

This group includes iohexol (Omnipaque), iopamidol (Isovue), and ioversol (Optiray). These agents are the most commonly used. Nonionic agents have three iodine atoms for each osmotically active particle (Figure 5.14). These agents are water soluble in a noncharged form (i.e., without an associated cation), and hence provide an equivalent amount of iodine as the ionic counterparts with lower osmolality.[4]

Iso-osmolar Contrast Media
Nonionic Dimers

This class of contrast agents has osmolality similar to that of plasma. They are nonionic dimers and contain six atoms of iodine per dimer and hence are ratio 6 agents (Figure 5.15). Iodixanol (Visipaque) is the only agent currently in this class. IOCM has the potential of causing fewer side effects in patients undergoing interventional procedures,[2] and its use is associated with fewer adverse cardiac events compared with LOCM. [2,3]

Although IOCM have been postulated to produce less cardioreflex activity, a recent randomized control trial found no differences in heart rate parameters between non-ionic LOCM and IOCM when using the same injection rate and total iodine dose.[4] There is also data suggesting a reduction in nephrotoxicity with this agent, although the magnitude of this benefit is still unresolved.[5] However, in the IMPACT study, a prospective trial failed to identify any difference in the incidence of contrast induced nephropathy between equal iodine doses of non-ionic LOCM and IOCM in patients with pre-existing stable chronically reduced kidney function.[6]

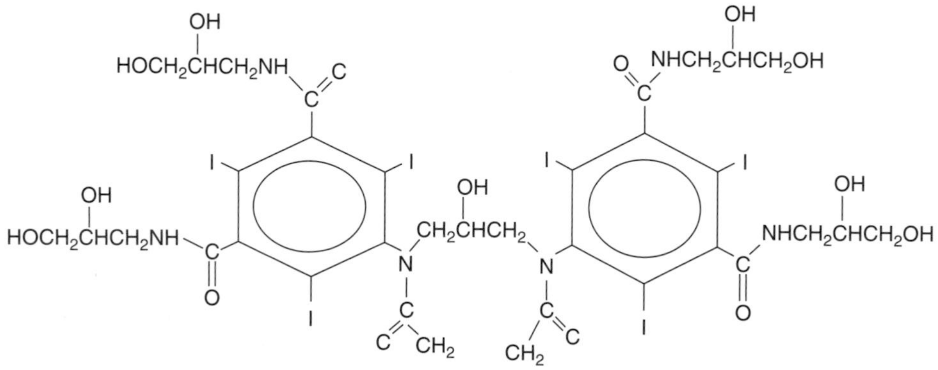

FIGURE 5.15 Nonionic dimmer, ratio 6 (6:1).

TABLE 5.9	Adverse Effects of Contrast Agents Can Be Grouped into the Following Categories		
Anaphylactoid Reaction	**Toxic Reaction**	**Delayed Reaction**	
Urticaria	Hot flushing sensation	Delayed skin reaction	
Angioedema	Nausea		
Bronchospasm	Arrhythmias		
Cardiovascular collapse	Renal failure	Flu-like syndrome	
	Skin damage from extravasation	Hyperthyroidism	
	Iodide mumps		

Adverse Effects of Contrast Agents

In general, nonionic compounds have fewer side effects as they do not dissociate into component molecules. The side effect profile is also dependent upon the osmolality of the compound, such that the hyperosmolar solutions have more side effects (Table 5.9).

Anaphylactoid reactions are immediate type reactions and are triggered by activation of basophils and macrophages in the lungs. This can cause rapid vasodilatation and circulatory collapse. It has also been reported that the intravenous use of iodinated contrast agents is associated with more events than the intra-arterial use, since the contrast given intravenously courses through lungs where it can trigger the cell activation. In distinction, late contrast reactions occur hours to days later.[7,8] The delayed skin reaction is a T-lymphocyte-mediated delayed hypersensitivity.[9]

Symptoms of delayed reactions may also resemble a flu-like syndrome and include fever, chills, nausea, vomiting, abdominal pain, fatigue, and congestion.[10]

Toxic reactions are caused by the inherent physical or chemical properties of contrast agents or the additives necessary for their stabilization. Most toxic effects are thought to result from the hyperosmolality of these agents.

Reaction to radiocontrast agents are classified according to their severity:

- Mild (grade I: single episode of emesis, nausea, sneezing, or vertigo)
- Moderate (grade II: hives, multiple episodes of emesis, fevers, or chills)
- Severe (grade III: clinical shock, bronchospasm, laryngospasm or edema, loss of consciousness, hypotension, hypertension, cardiac arrhythmias, angioedema, or pulmonary edema)

The reported incidence of severe reactions is about 1:1000,[11,12] and of deaths, about 1:12,000 to 1:75,000.[10,11]

Iodide mumps is an uncommon complication of intravascular administration of iodinated contrast.[13] The reaction arises as an acute inflammatory swelling of the submandibular, sublingual, or parotid glands.

Iodide mumps have been reported after administration of high- and low-osmolar iodide contrast media.[14] The mechanism of response is unclear and could be related to a toxic accumulation of iodide in the salivary glands, as suggested by a high proportion of patients with renal impairment.[15] No life-threatening reaction has been reported, and remission occurs spontaneously within a few days. Current therapy is supportive; however, early hemodialysis may shorten the duration of swelling in patients with renal failure.[16]

Contrast Reaction Prophylaxis

There is little cross-reactivity between the different classes of the radiocontrast agents. If a patient had a prior reaction to a contrast agent, obtaining a careful history is helpful in this regard. If the patient's reaction occurred in the United States before 1985, a nonionic, low-osmolality agent could not have been used, so one could be used now. If the reaction occurred before 1997, iodixanol, the nonionic isotonic dimer, was not available, so it could be substituted.

The presence of a history of multiple severe allergies and allergies to eggs and peanut butter does increase the risk of a reaction following contrast agent injection, but only by a very small percentage.[17] In the past, many thought that an allergy to shellfish was a predictor of an increased risk of a reaction to a contrast agent, presumably because both shellfish and contrast agents contain iodine. Such a relationship is not correct. Organic iodide as found in shellfish is an essential element (i.e., I_2 vs. I^-), so individuals cannot be allergic to it.

The following premedication protocol has been recommended for use in patients with a history of prior moderate or severe contrast reactions:

Methylprednisolone (one 32-mg tablet at 12 hours and 2 hours before the study), or Prednisone (one 50-mg tablet at 13 hours, 7 hours, and 1 hour before the study).[18]

The physician may also consider adding the following though it is unclear whether these medications alter the incidence of developing a moderate or severe contrast reaction:

An H_1 blocker such as diphenhydramine (one 50-mg tablet 1 hour before the study), and An H_2 blocker (optional) such as cimetidine (Tagamet), one 300-mg tablet 1 hour before the study, or ranitidine (Zantac), one 50-mg tablet 1 hour before the study.[19]

The LOCM and IOCM have reduced the incidence of acute allergic-like phenomena accompanying angiography; however, delayed reactions, predominantly rash, may occur hours to days after exposure. Some of these are associated with antibody responses to the particular contrast (or possibly an additive).[7,20] Symptoms of delayed reactions (nausea, vomiting, abdominal pain, fluid overload, and fatigue) usually resolve spontaneously and require only supportive management.

Treatment of Anaphylactoid Reactions

The principles of advanced cardiac life support should be followed in the treatment of anaphylactic reactions to contrast media. Stabilization of the patient's airway, cardiac function, and blood pressure is the fundamental element of treating anaphylactic reactions. Intravenous fluid bolus with 250–500 mL of normal saline should be given to patients with hypotension and/or shock. In patients who develop bronchospasm, laryngeal edema, or severe urticaria or angioedema, epinephrine should be administered immediately (0.3–0.5 mg subcutaneously every 10–20 minutes).

Antihistamine therapy is considered adjunctive to epinephrine. Diphenhydramine (Benadryl) 25–50 mg should be given intravenously.

Bronchospasm that has not responded to subcutaneous epinephrine should be treated with inhaled β2-adrenergic agonists such as albuterol.

Corticosteroids do not have an immediate effect on anaphylaxis; however, administer them early to prevent a potential late-phase reaction (biphasic anaphylaxis). Hydrocortisone, 50 mg, or 50 mg of methylprednisolone can be given intravenously.

Contrast-Induced Nephropathy

The most commonly used definition of contrast-induced nephropathy (CIN) is a rise in the serum creatinine of 0.5 mg/dL.[23] Occasionally, a 1 mg/dL rise in the scrum creatinine or a 25% increase in the serum creatinine has been used.[23–25]

Pathophysiology and Risk Factors for CIN

The specific cause for contrast-induced nephropathy is not known, but it is characterized by acute tubular necrosis. Contrast-induced nephropathy results from injury to the renal medulla caused by a combination of reduced renal blood flow, osmotic shift of fluid into the distal tubules, and direct renal tubular toxicity.[24] Worsening of renal function may occur after contrast-agent administration in 13%–20% of patients, and is highest in those with prior renal insufficiency, diabetes mellitus, dehydration before the procedure, chronic heart failure, large amount of contrast, and with recent (<48-hour) contrast exposure.[26–29]

The rise in the serum creatinine usually does not occur until 24–48 hours following contrast exposure, and the peak rise in serum creatinine occurs 4–5 days after contrast exposure. Therefore, unless systematic testing is used, many episodes of mild contrast-induced nephropathy may go undetected.

Prevention of Contrast-Induced Nephropathy

Hydration

The risk of contrast-induced nephropathy may be lessened with fluid administration before the procedure.[24,30,31] With many protocols published but no one specific regimen identified, it is strongly recommended to administer parenterally a total of at least 1 L of isotonic saline beginning at least 3 hours before and continuing at least 6–8 hours after the procedure. Initial infusion rates of 100–150 mL per hour are recommended with adjustment post procedure as clinically indicated. Appropriate caution should be applied for the patient with known reduced left ventricular function or congestive heart failure. To accomplish this regimen, outpatients should be scheduled for early arrival or later procedure times; prior-day admission may be required in selected patients.[32]

Sodium Bicarbonate

The use of isotonic sodium bicarbonate has been demonstrated in one study to be marginally superior to isotonic sodium chloride (saline) in preventing CIN in high-risk patients.[33] In this study, patients received either sodium chloride or sodium bicarbonate, both as 154-mEq/L infusions (3 mL/kg during the hour before contrast administration, and 1 mL/kg during and for 6 hours after the procedure). Although additional studies are needed, these data suggest that a modified regimen with sodium bicarbonate may be effective in high-risk patients.

Avoid/Hold Nephrotoxic Medications

Review patients' medications and withhold, as clinically appropriate, potentially nephrotoxic drugs, including aminoglycoside antibiotics, anti-rejection medications, and nonsteroidal anti-inflammatory drugs (NSAIDs).

Angiotensin-converting enzyme inhibitor therapy may be continued, but neither initiating nor changing dose should be considered until the patient is safely past the risk period for CIN.[33]

N-Acetylcysteine

Relying on the assumption that reactive oxygen species might be involved in the pathogenesis of CIN, N-acetylcysteine (NAC) has been evaluated by several studies. Six hundred milligrams orally, twice daily the day before and the day of contrast administration in patients with underlying renal insufficiency reduced the incidence of contrast-induced nephropathy in some studies.[34,35] Several other trials designed to confirm the benefit of NAC in patients with chronic renal insufficiency undergoing angiography have provided conflicting results.[36,37]

Hemodialysis and Hemofiltration

Hemodialysis has been shown to remove radiographic contrast media but not to prevent CIN.[38] Hemofiltration allows increased hemodynamic stability compared with hemodialysis, while permitting 10–15 times the usual hydration without adding intravascular volume. Though promising in small studies, hemofiltration is invasive and logistically complex. It will need to be established in larger trials before it can be widely recommended.[39]

Contrast Volume

Total case contrast volume is a risk factor for CIN.[23] Intuitively, the less amount of contrast administered, the lower the risk for CIN. In coronary CTA the scan is acquired in a single breath hold during comfortable inspiration and starts with the injection of a contrast agent with a high concentration of iodine (300–400 mg/mL) at a high flow rate (4–6 mL/s).[40] The total volume of contrast agent depends on the scan length. On average, in a 16-slice CT scanner about 70–100 mL is used, and in a 64-slice CT scanner 50–80 mL of contrast is used.[40] In a study by Freeman, contrast doses above 5 cc × body weight (kg)/SCr were associated with a need for dialysis, and unadjusted contrast dose was not a univariate predictor of contrast induced dialysis.[41]

Diabetic patients with underlying renal insufficiency (serum creatinine ≥1.5) may also benefit from the use of the IOCM as compared to LOCM.[9]

Many agents studied have not shown a consistent benefit in reducing the incidence of CIN when compared to volume repletion alone. These include mannitol,[42] post-procedural diuretics,[9] dopamine,[43] fenoldopam,[44] atrial natriuretic peptide,[45] and calcium channel blockers.[46]

It should be emphasized that even the best current radiographic contrast agents still have complications in terms of allergic reactions and kidney injury. The volume of contrast that may be used in a given procedure is thus limited, and patients with pre-procedure risk factors need aggressive pre-procedure hydration, and possibly a renoprotective drug regimen.

REFERENCES

1. Zuckerman LS, Frichliing TD, Wolf NM, et al. Effect of calcium binding additives on ventricular fibrillation and repolarization changes during coronary angiography. *J Am Coll Cardiol.* 1987; 10:1249.
2. Bertrand ME, Esplugas E, Piessens J, Rasch W. Influence of a nonionic, iso-osmolar contrast medium (iodixanol) versus an ionic, low osmolar contrast medium (ioxaglate) on major adverse cardiac events in patients undergoing percutaneous transluminal coronary angioplasty: A multicenter, randomized, double blind study. Visipaque in Percutaneous Transluminal Coronary Angioplasty VIP Trial Investigators. *Circulation.* 2000; 101:131–136.
3. Piao ZE, Murdock DK, Hwang MH, et al. Hemodynamic abnormalities during coronary angiography: Comparison of Hypaque 76, Hexabrix, and Omnipaque-350. *Cathet Cardiovasc Diagn.* 1989; 16:149.
4. Sahani DV, Soulez G, Chen K, et al. A Comparison of the Efficacy and Safety of Iopamidol-370 and Iodixanol-320 in Patients Undergoing Multidetector-Row Computed Tomography. *Investigative Radiology.* 2007; 42:856–861.
5. Grines CL, Schreiber TL, Savas V, et al. A randomized trial of low osmolar ionic versus nonionic contrast media in patients with myocardial infarction or unstable angina undergoing percutaneous transluminal coronary angioplasty. *J Am Coll Cardiol.* 1996; 27:1381–1386.
6. Barrett BJ, Katzberg RW, Thomsen HS, et al for the IMPACT Study Investigators. Contrast Induced Nephropathy in Patients with Chronic Kidney Disease Undergoing Computed Tomography: A Double-blind Comparison of Iodixanol and Iopamidol. *Investigative Radiol.* 2006; 41:815–821.
7. Davidson CJ, Laskey WK, Hermiller JB, et al. Randomized trial of contrast media utilization in high-risk PTCA: The COURT trial. *Circulation.* 2000; 101:2172–2177.
8. Lasser EC, Berry CC, Talner LB, et al. Pretreatment with corticosteroids to alleviate reactions to intravenous contrast material. *N Engl J Med.* 1987; 317:845–849.

9. Aspelin P, Aubry P, Fransson SG, et al. Nephrotoxic effects in high-risk patients undergoing angiography (iodixanol). *N Engl J Med.* 2003; 348:491–499.

10. Pedersen SH, Svaland MG, Reiss AL, Andrew E. Late allergy-like reactions following vascular administration of radiography contrast media. *Acta Radiol.* 1998; 39:344–348.

11. Christiansen C, Pichler WJ, Skotland T. Delayed allergy-like reactions to X-ray contrast media: mechanistic considerations. *Eur Radiol.* 2000; 10;1965–1975.

12. Dewachter, et al. Anti-inflammatory and anti-allergy agents. 2006 May; 5(2):105–117(13).

13. Maddox TG. *Am Fam Physician.* Adverse reactions to contrast material: recognition, prevention, and treatment. 2002; 66:1229–1234.

14. Ansell G, Tweedie MCK, West CR, Evans P, Couch L. The current status of reactions to intravenous contrast media. *Invest Radiol.* 1980; 15(suppl):S32–S39.

15. Shehadi WH, Toniolo G. Adverse reactions to contrast media: A report from the Committee on Safety of Contrast Media of the International Society of Radiology. Radiology. 1980; 137:299–302.

16. Sussman RM, Miller J. Iodide mumps after intravenous urography. *N Engl J Med.* 1956; 255:433–434.

17. Christensen J. Iodide mumps after intravascular administration of a nonionic contrast medium. Case report and review of the literature. *Acta Radiol.* 1995; 36:82–84.

18. Harris PF, Sanchez JF, Mode DG. Iodide mumps. *JAMA.* 1970; 213:2271–2272.

19. Kalaria VG, Porsche R, Ong LS. Iodide mumps: Acute sialadenitis after contrast administration for angioplasty. *Circulation.* 2001; 104:2384.

20. Bettmann MA, Heeren T, Greenfield A, Goudey C. Adverse events with radiographic contrast agents: Results of the SCVIR Contrast Agent Registry. *Radiology.* 1997; 203:611–620.

21. Cohan RH, Ellis JH. Iodinated contrast material in uroradiology. Choice of agent and management of complications. *Urol Clin North Am.* 1997; 24:471–491.

22. Kelly JF, Patterson R, Lieberman P, Mathison DA, Stevenson DD. Radiographic contrast media studies in high risk patients. *J Allergy Clin Immunol.* 1978; 62;181–184.

23. Davidson CJ, Laskey WK, Hermiller JB, et al. Randomized trial of contrast media utilization in high-risk PTCA: The COURT trial. *Circulation.* 2000; 101:2172–2177.

24. Mehran R, Aymong ED, Nikolsky E, et al. A simple risk score for prediction of contrast-induced nephropathy after percutaneous coronary intervention: Development and initial validation. *J Am Coll Cardiol.* 2004; 44:1393–1399.

25. Baker CS. Prevention of radiocontrast-induced nephropathy. Catheter Cardiovasc Interv. 2003; 58:532–538.

26. Adair W, Harris K. Using estimated GFR values to identify patients at risk from iodinated contrast induced nephropathy. *Clinical Radiol.* 2006; 61(8):714–715.

27. Baker CS. Prevention of radiocontrast-induced nephropathy. *Catheter Cardiovasc Interv.* 2003; 58:532–538.

28. Agrawal M, Stouffer GA. Cardiology Grand Rounds from The University of North Carolina at Chapel Hill. Contrast induced nephropathy after angiography. *Am J Med Sci.* 2002; 323:252–258.

29. Gomes VO, Blaya P, Poli de Figueiredo CE, Manfroi W, Caramori P. Contrast-media induced nephropathy in patients undergoing coronary angiography. *J Invasive Cardiol.* 2003; 15:304–310.

30. Huber W, Schipek C, Ilgmann K, et al. Effectiveness of theophylline prophylaxis of renal impairment after coronary angiography in patients with chronic renal insufficiency. *Am J Cardiol.* 2003; 91:1157–1162.

31. Solomon R. Radiocontrast-induced nephropathy. *Semin Nephrol.* 1998; 18:551–557.

32. Stevens MA, McCullough PA, Tobin KJ, et al. A prospective randomized trial of prevention measures in patients at high risk for contrast nephropathy: Results of the PRINCE Study. Prevention of Radiocontrast Induced Nephropathy Clinical Evaluation. *J Am Coll Cardiol.* 1999; 33:403–411.

33. Mueller C, Buerkle G, Buettner HJ, et al. Prevention of contrast media-associated nephropathy: Randomized comparison of 2 hydration regimens in 1620 patients undergoing coronary angioplasty. *Arch Intern Med.* 2002; 162:329–336.

34. Schwieger MJ, et al. *Cathet Cardiovasc Interv.* 2007; 69(1):135–140.

35. Merten GJ, Burgess WP, Gray LV, et al. Prevention of contrast-induced nephropathy with sodium bicarbonate: A randomized controlled trial. *JAMA.* 2004; 291:2328–2334.

36. Tepel M, van der Giet M, Schwarzfeld C, Laufer U, Liermann D, Zidek W. Prevention of radiographic-contrast-agent-induced reductions in renal function by acetylcysteine. *N Engl J Med.* 2000; 343:180–184.

37. Baker CS, Wragg A, Kumar S, De Palma R, Baker LR, Knight CJ. A rapid protocol for the prevention of contrast-induced renal dysfunction: The RAPPID study. *J Am Coll Cardiol.* 2003; 41:2114–2118.

38. Durham JD, Caputo C, et al. A rondomized controlled trial of N-acetylcysteine to prevent contrast nephropathy in cardiac angiography. *Kidney Int.* 2002; 62:2202–2207.

39. Boccalandro F, Ahmad M, et al. Oral acetylcysteine does not protect renal funtion from moderate to high doses of intravenous radiographic contrast. *Cathet Cardiovasc Interv.* 2003; 58:336–341.

40. Sterner G, Frennby B, Kurkus K, Nyman U. Does post-angiographic hemodialysis reduce the risk of contrast medium nephropathy? Scand *J Urol Nephrol.* 2000; 34:323–326.

41. Marenzi G, Marana I, Lauri G, et al. The prevention of radiocontrast-agent-induced nephropathy by hemofiltration. *N Engl J Med.* 2003; 349:1333–1340.

42. Hoffman U, et al. Coronary CT angiography. *J Nucl Med.* 2006; 47(5):797–806.

43. Freeman RV, O'Donnell M, Share D, et al. Nephropathy requiring dialysis after percutaneous coronary intervention and the critical role of an adjusted contrast dose. *Am J Cardiol.* 2002; 90:1068–1073.

44. Aspelin P, Aubry P, Fransson SG, et al. Nephrotoxic effects in high-risk patients undergoing angiography (iodixanol). *N Engl J Med.* 2003; 348:491–499.

45. Solomon R, Werner C, Mann D, D'Elia J, Silva P. Effects of saline, mannitol, and furosemide to prevent acute decreases in renal function induced by radiocontrast agents. *N Engl J Med.* 1994; 331:1416–1420.

46. Gare M, Haviv YS, Ben-Yehuda A, et al. The renal effect of low-dose dopamine in high-risk patients undergoing coronary angiography. *J Am Coll Cardiol.* 1999; 34:1682–1688.

47. Stone GW, McCullough PA, Tumlin JA, et al. Fenoldopam mesylate for the prevention of contrast-induced nephropathy: A randomized controlled trial. *JAMA.* 2003; 290:2284–2291.

48. Kurnik BR, Allgren RL, Genter FC, et al. Prospective study of atrial natriuretic peptide for the prevention of radiocontrast-induced nephropathy. *Am J Kidney Dis.* 1998; 31:674–680.

49. Khoury Z, Schlicht JR, Como J, et al. The effect of prophylactic nifedipine on renal function in patients administered contrast media. *Pharacotherapy.* 1995; 15:59–65.

CHAPTER 6

Kim Arellano-Villarreal and Raymond Q. Migrino

Cardiac Magnetic Resonance Imaging in Coronary Artery Disease

Cardiac magnetic resonance imaging (CMR) is an established modality in the comprehensive assessment of coronary artery disease. The advantages of CMR over other imaging modalities include high spatial resolution, lack of exposure to ionizing radiation, ability to acquire unlimited imaging planes, and the ability to characterize tissues. Perhaps most importantly is its versatility in the assessment of clinical questions relevant to ischemic heart disease, ranging from myocardial function, perfusion, viability, coronary stenosis, and sequelae of myocardial infarct, including presence of left ventricular aneurysm or pseudoaneurysm, thrombus, and valve dysfunction.

Basic Principles, Image Acquisition, and Safety

Cardiac magnetic resonance imaging is based on the exploitation of the magnetization properties of hydrogen protons to acquire images. In the presence of the powerful magnetic field provided by the MRI scanner, frequently 1.5 Tesla (with increasing use of 3 Tesla), the body's protons align with the magnetic field with fewer aligned in the direction opposite the external magnetic field; a net magnetization is created with precession (spin) of protons in the direction of the external field. To create an image, brief external radiofrequency pulses at a resonant frequency dependent on the proton's gyromagnetic ratio (an intrinsic property of the proton) and magnetic field strength are applied. The radiofrequency pulse causes the hydrogen protons to absorb energy, causing disruption of their net magnetization. Once the radiofrequency pulse is turned off, the protons return to their original alignment to the external magnetic field. Receiver coils on the surface of the body detect the changes in magnetization that occur as the protons realign and convert it into electrical signals that form the basis of MRI images. Spatial localization of the signal is accomplished using gradient coils that create subtle differences in regional resonant frequency in three dimensions. Radiofrequency pulses are repeated until enough signals are acquired to form an image.

The two basic pulse sequences in CMR are "dark blood" or spin echo sequence, where the blood pool appears dark against a bright myocardium, and "bright blood" or gradient echo sequence (the most frequently used is the steady state free precession gradient echo), where the blood pool appears bright against a dark myocardium (Figure 6.1). In general, dark blood imaging is used for structural evaluation, and bright blood imaging (with the use of cine, or dynamic, imaging) is used for functional evaluation.

Unlike other MRI techniques, central to cardiac imaging is the need for electrocardiographic (ECG) gating because of cardiac motion. Because of the low signal of the precessing protons, multiple radiofrequency pulses and signal acquisitions are needed to form an image, frequently requiring multiple heartbeats acquired in one breath hold. Thus, unlike echocardiography, most MRI sequences rely on images averaged over several heart beats and are not acquired in real time. Although real time imaging currently exists in CMR, the temporal resolution required for such acquisition comes at the expense of spatial resolution, thus real time

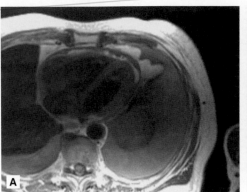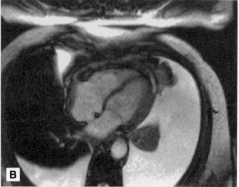

FIGURE 6.1 Cardiac magnetic resonance imaging pulse sequences. (*A*) Spin echo ("black blood") imaging in the axial plane in the mid-ventricle. Note the suppression of blood pool signal and clear delineation of myocardial region. There is a large left pleural effusion and small right pleural effusion. (*B*) Gradient echo ("bright blood") imaging. This is a steady state free precession sequence showing bright blood pool. Note the contrast between the blood pool and the myocardium. This sequence is frequently used for cine functional imaging.

imaging is not frequently used in most diagnostic sequences. Cardiac motion in most protocols is compensated for with the use of ECG gating, and respiratory motion is addressed by acquiring images while the patient is holding a breath.

Magnetic resonance imaging is one of the safest noninvasive imaging modalities and does not involve ionizing radiation. The only absolute contraindication to CMR involves patients with ferromagnetic materials such as pacemakers, defibrillators, cerebral aneurysm clips, etc. Another contraindication is severe claustrophobia. Patients with prosthetic cardiac valves (except for older models of ball and cage design with ferromagnetic materials) and established cardiac stents are deemed safe for CMR. A relative contraindication for CMR includes pregnancy, as potential risks to the fetus are not well established. Recently, there have been isolated and rare reports about the development of nephrogenic systemic fibrosis, manifesting as swelling and tightening of the skin in patients with moderate to end-stage renal dysfunction who received gadolinium-based contrast agents. Until this is further studied, there is a Food and Drug Administration advisory against the use of gadolinium agents in patients with significant renal dysfunction. For more complete information on MRI safety, an excellent resource is www.mrisafety.com.

Evaluation of Ventricular Size and Function

Cardiac magnetic resonance imaging is superior to other modalities for quantification of ventricular size and function, and is deemed the gold standard noninvasive modality to measure these parameters. It has high spatial resolution, unlimited imaging planes, and image quality is not affected by body habitus. Ventricular volume and function is derived using the stacked disc method (modified Simpson's method), a true volumetric measure that does not rely on geometric assumptions that may not be applicable to certain ventricular shapes, such as dilated left ventricles, or the many variations of normal right ventricular shape (Figure 6.2). Compared with echocardiography, CMR had superior interstudy reproducibility in the assessment of ventricular volumes, function, and masses in normal and diseased hearts.[1] The steady-state free precession gradient echo is the pulse sequence of choice for evaluating ventricular function because of the excellent contrast between ventricular blood pool and cardiac

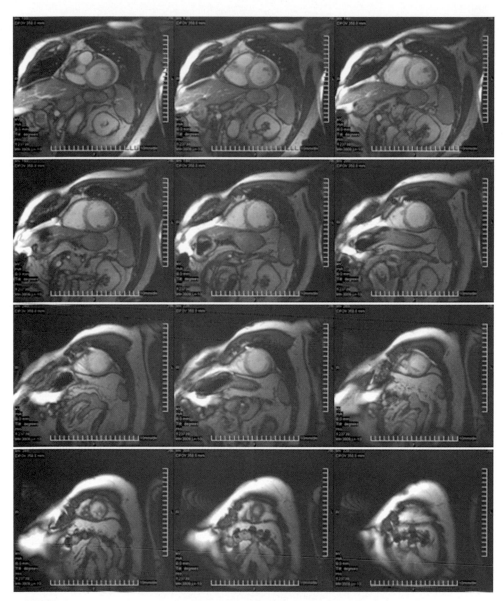

FIGURE 6.2   Multislice short axis evaluation of the left and right ventricular function. Sequential short axis thin slices of the ventricles are obtained on cine steady-state free precession. Using manual or semiauto-mated methods of border detection, endocardial border is traced throughout the cardiac cycle. Ventricular volumes and ejection fraction are calculated using modified Simpson's method (stacked disc method).

muscle. Ventricular volumes and ejection fractions can be calculated with the use of various commercially available analysis software packages using both manual or automated endocardial border detection. Established normal values are presented in Table 6.1.[2]

Similar to echocardiography and nuclear methods, regional wall motion abnormalities are assessed and reported using the standard 16- or 17-segment model. In addition to steady-state free precession sequence, myocardial tagging can also be used to evaluate cardiac motion (Figure 6.3). With this technique, spatial saturation bands are applied during the pulse sequence, resulting in dark lines or a crosshatched grid pattern that is superimposed on the

TABLE 6.1	Normal Ventricular Parameters Using Cardiac Magnetic Resonance Imaging		
	All	**Males**	**Females**
LVEDV (mL)	121 (55–187)	136 (77–195)	96 (52–141)
LVESV (mL)	40 (13–67)	45 (19–72)	32 (13–51)
LVEF (%)	67 (57–78)	67 (57–78)	67 (57–78)
RVEDV (mL)	138 (59–217)	157 (88–227)	106 (58–154)
RVESV (mL)	54 (12–96)	63 (23–103)	40 (12–68)
RVEF (%)	61 (47–76)	60 (47–74)	63 (47–80)
LV mass (g)	104 (44–150)	117 (75–159)	82 (46–119)
LVEDVI (mL/m^2)	66 (44–89)	69 (47–92)	61 (41–81)
RVEDVI (mL/m^2)	75 (49–101)	80 (55–105)	67 (48–87)
LVMI (g/m^2)	87 (64–109)	91 (70–113)	79 (63–95)

Values expressed as mean (95% confidence interval).
LVEDV and RVEDV, left and right ventricular end-diastolic volume; LVESV and RVESV, left and right end-systolic volume; LVEF and RVEF, left and right ventricular ejection fraction; LVEDVI and RVEDVI, left and right ventricular end-diastolic volume index; LVM and LVMI, left ventricular mass and mass index
Lorenz CH, Walker ES, Morgan VL, et al. Normal human right and left ventricular mass, systolic function, and gender differences by cine magnetic resonance imaging. *J Cardiovasc Magn Reson.* 1999; 1:7–21.

ventricular myocardium throughout the cardiac cycle. Deformation of the tag lines during ventricular contraction may aid in evaluation of normal or abnormal regional wall motion. Lack of deformation of the tag lines suggests a region of nonfunctioning myocardium. Although now infrequently used for assessment of regional function, tagged cine MRI can be used for calculation of regional strain.

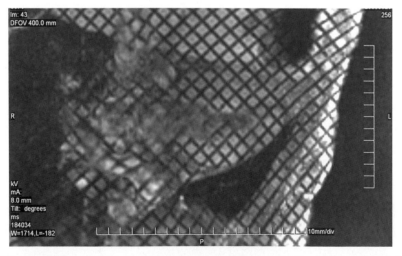

FIGURE 6.3 Tagged cine gradient echo of the left ventricle in the two-chamber (oblique sagittal) view. The dark grids are saturation bands that "tag" the myocardium during the cardiac cycle. This is used to evaluate regional myocardial function as well as local deformation.

Ischemia Evaluation

There is increasing use of CMR for ischemia evaluation. There are two methods of assessing myocardial ischemia: (1) perfusion imaging using first-pass gadolinium contrast at rest and following administration of coronary vasodilators (Adenosine or dipyridamole), or (2) assessment of contractile reserve following inotropic stimulation with dobutamine.

A unique challenge to performing stress evaluation in the MRI suite relates to the magnetic environment. Unlike other methods, ECG changes cannot be interpreted inside the magnet because of the "magneto hydrodynamic effect." High flow velocities in the great vessels during systole in the presence of a high magnetic field create electrical signals that alter the underlying ECG signal, especially in the ST segment that corresponds in timing to the greatest flow. Thus, ECG monitoring can only reliably assess heart rate but not ischemic change. Also, confinement within the MRI scanner may present additional challenges both to the patient as well as the supervising staff. Overall, however, the safety and efficacy of CMR for ischemia evaluation are well established.

Perfusion Stress MRI

Although dipyridamole can be used for ischemia imaging, most centers use Adenosine because of its extremely short half-life (<10 seconds) and better patient tolerance. Adenosine causes coronary vasodilation and recruitment of capillary beds. A myocardial territory supplied by a coronary artery without significant stenosis increases perfusion several-fold by recruitment of additional capillary beds following Adenosine infusion. Myocardium supplied by a coronary artery with significant stenosis, on the other hand, has adapted to this flow limitation with recruitment of available capillary beds at rest to maintain perfusion; Adenosine infusion results in significantly lower increment of capillary bed recruitment compared to territories without coronary stenosis. This leads to relative reduction of flow in areas supplied by coronary arteries with significant stenoses. The patient receives 2–3 minutes of Adenosine infusion (140 µg/kg per minute), frequently initiated with the patient just outside the scanner bore for closer monitoring by the nursing personnel. The patient is then positioned inside the scanner and gadolinium-DTPA (0.05–0.2 mmol/kg) is rapidly infused and first pass imaging is performed using a gradient echo pulse sequence on multiple short axis slices of the left ventricle performed during a breath hold. Normal myocardium will show a "blush" of bright signal throughout the cardiac cycle, whereas ischemic or infarcted myocardium will show a persistent dark signal, either subendocardial or transmural in location (Figure 6.4). To differentiate between ischemic and infarcted myocardium, rest perfusion imaging without Adenosine is performed (Table 6.2). Abnormal areas following Adenosine infusion that have normal resting perfusion are considered ischemic. If the signal abnormality persists, this area is either infarcted (verified by presence of delayed enhancement) or the signal abnormality is an artifact (if there is no delayed enhancement). However, resting ischemia, although rare, may also present with low signal intensity during Adenosine infusion and rest, and with no delayed enhancement. Assessment of the patient's clinical status is necessary to determine in this rare case if this is resting ischemia or artifact.

Image interpretation is usually qualitative, with rest and post Adenosine images evaluated side by side. Semiquantitative and quantitative methods have been developed, but these methods have yet to be widely validated in the clinical setting and are still largely in the realm of research applications. Furthermore, unlike positron emission tomography (PET)-based perfusion imaging, CMR imaging cannot directly and accurately measure myocardial blood flow, and quantitative methods using myocardial signal-time curves make the assumption that the signal is proportional to underlying myocardial blood flow.

Adenosine stress CMR has good sensitivity and specificity in detecting significant coronary artery disease (Table 6.3) and is comparable to conventional nuclear methods. However,

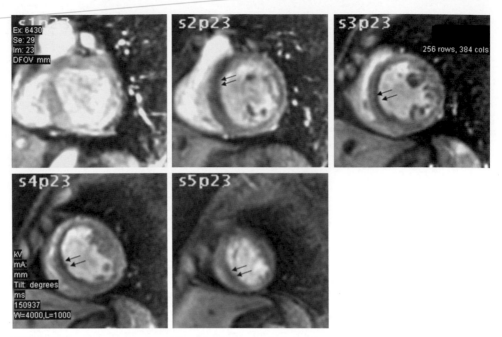

FIGURE 6.4 First pass perfusion CMR study. Short axis slices showing resting perfusion following gadolinium injection. There is reduced subendocardial perfusion in the base to distal anteroseptum and inferoseptum and apical inferoseptum (*arrows*). This signifies subendocardial scar or fixed defect. To differentiate scar or fixed defect from artifact, gadolinium delayed enhancement would be present in these regions in myocardial scar. Artifact would not show delayed enhancement.

because CMR has superior spatial resolution compared to single photon emission computed tomography (SPECT), subendocardial disease can be detected. Other advantages of CMR over SPECT are the lack of ionizing radiation and shorter total duration of the test. In addition, because MRI uses first pass perfusion, imaging can be started after achievement of maximal Adenosine-induced vasodilation, usually 2 minutes following infusion. In contrast,

TABLE 6.2	Asssessment of Ischemia, Infarction/scar, and Viability of Myocardial Segments in Cardiac Magnetic Resonance Imaging		
	Ischemia	**Infarcted, Not Viable**	**Infarcted but Viable**
Adenosine stress CMR			
Rest perfusion	Normal signal	Signal loss	Signal loss
Post Adenosine perfusion	Signal loss	Signal loss	Signal loss
Delayed enhancement	None	>50%	<50%
Dobutamine stress CMR			
Rest wall motion	Normal	Abnormal	Abnormal
Post dobutamine wall motion	Abnormal	Abnormal	Improvement at low dose, worsening at high dose
Delayed enhancement	None	>50%	<50%

CMR, cardiac magnetic resonance imaging

TABLE 6.3	Sensitivity and Specificity of Perfusion and Dobutamine CMR for Diagnosis of Coronary Artery Disease			
Reference	**n**	**Technique**	**Sensitivity**	**Specificity**
3 (Klem 2006)	92	Perf+DE	89	84
4 (Positano 2006)	32	Perf	88	86
5 (Sakuma 2005)	48	Perf	81	68
6 (Wolff 2004)	99	Perf	93	75
7 (Nagel 2003)	90	Perf	88	90
8 (Ishida 2003)	104	Perf	90	85
9 (Schwitter 2001)	66	Perf	87	85
10 (Nagel 1999)	208	Dobutamine	86	86

SPECT-based imaging relies on intracellular uptake of radiotracer, and requires a longer infusion of Adenosine, frequently 4–6 minutes. Other advantages of CMR include functional and morphological evaluation of the heart.

Contraindications to the use of Adenosine include second- or third-degree heart block, sinus node disease, and obstructive pulmonary disease such as asthma or chronic obstructive pulmonary disease.

Dobutamine Stress CMR

Like dobutamine stress echocardiography, dobutamine stress CMR relies on inotropic stimulation to induce wall motion abnormality in myocardial territories supplied by an epicardial coronary artery with significant stenosis (Table 6.2). Similar dosing is used with a progressive increase from 5–10 and up to 40 µg/kg per minute in 3-minute intervals. The aim is to increase the heart rate to greater than 85% of maximum predicted heart rate. Augmentation of heart rate response with atropine can be used to reach this target level, if needed. Serial cardiac cines are acquired at rest and at different dosing intervals in multiple slices from base to apex to assess for regional or global wall motion abnormalities.

Myocardial ischemia is suggested by resting normal segment wall motion and induced wall motion abnormality (hypokinesia, akinesia, or dyskinesia) with dobutamine infusion. Balanced global ischemia is suggested by ventricular dilatation accompanied by either global hypokinesia or seemingly preserved segmental wall motion following dobutamine infusion. Scar or infarction is suggested by resting wall motion abnormality that persists or worsens with dobutamine infusion.

Because of the inability to use the ECG to reliably detect ischemia while the patient is in the scanner, operators rely on immediate, real-time assessment of wall motion abnormality as well as the patient's status to determine whether to proceed or stop the test. Compared to the Adenosine stress test, dobutamine stress MRI entails a longer examination time inside the magnet, necessitates real-time image interpretation for inducible ischemia, and has the potential for inotropic-induced ventricular arrhythmias. However, the safety of dobutamine stress CMR has been established and the sensitivity and specificity of this modality (Table 6.3) compares favorably with echo and SPECT-based evaluation of coronary artery disease.

An additional advantage of dobutamine stress CMR is the evaluation of myocardial viability. Hypoperfused but viable myocardium resulting from flow limiting coronary stenosis may appear hypocontractile at rest. With low dose dobutamine (2.5–5 µg/kg per minute) these viable myocytes demonstrate contractile reserve in the presence of the inotropic agent with improvement in segmental wall motion. However, at higher dobutamine doses, the restricted perfusion does not allow sufficient blood flow, leading to reduced contractility. This biphasic response is a sign of segmental myocardial viability. This functional evaluation of viability complements the structural evaluation of viability using delayed enhancement imaging.

Dobutamine use is contraindicated in idiopathic hypertrophic subaortic stenosis, severe arterial hypertension, and known ventricular tachycardia.

Coronary Stenosis Evaluation

Coronary magnetic resonance angiography has been shown to detect significant coronary artery disease with great accuracy. In a multicenter trial involving 109 subjects, CMR had 100% sensitivity, 85% specificity, and 100% negative predictive value for diagnosing left main or three-vessel disease with 81% negative predictive value for any coronary artery disease.[11] However, coronary angiography has not been established as a routine clinical procedure because of existing limitations to the technique. One is the inability to evaluate about 15% of proximal and middle epicardial coronary artery segments, and the other is the duration of time of the examination. Improvements in navigator sequences (to correct for respiratory and cardiac motion), software (pulse sequence, parallel imaging, whole heart imaging), and hardware (multichannel coils, faster gradient performance) are being developed to make coronary angiography more clinically useful. The use of CMR is tempered currently by the relative ease of acquisition using multidetector computed tomography techniques whereby image acquisition is completed in less than half a minute, with comparable accuracy in coronary stenosis detection.

Coronary angiography with CMR is currently most commonly applied toward noninvasive detection of anomalous origin of coronary arteries (Figure 6.5). The lack of ionizing radiation, as well as three-dimensional visualization of adjacent structures, are advantages of CMR over invasive coronary as well as computed tomography angiography.

FIGURE 6.5 Anomalous origin of the right coronary artery from the left coronary sinus. Steady-state free precession gradient echo image shows the right coronary artery (*) anomalous origin and interarterial course between the aorta and the pulmonary artery. Ao, aorta; PA, pulmonary artery.

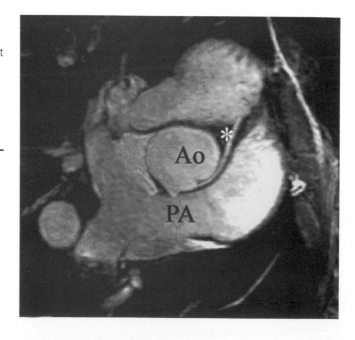

Infarct Imaging and Viability Assessment

Myocardial Viability

Distinguishing between viable and nonviable myocardium (infarct or scar) is important as it carries prognostic and therapeutic implications. A myocardial segment that is akinetic or severely hypokinetic may be nonviable, but it may also represent viable myocardium that is hibernating or stunned. While function cannot be restored to nonviable tissue, hibernating or stunned myocardium may recover function after revascularization. Identification of viable myocardium is useful in analyzing which patients will have improved left ventricular function and survival after cardiac revascularization.

The acceptance of MRI as an imaging tool accelerated with the introduction of post-gadolinium delayed enhancement protocols that provided, for the first time, infarct imaging with high spatial resolution that is highly correlated with histology assessment.

Gadolinium-DTPA is an extracellular contrast agent that shortens T1 relaxation in adjacent tissues, leading to higher tissue signal intensity. Following injection, areas of infarct or scar caused by cellular necrosis, inflammation, or fibrosis have increased volume of distribution of gadolinium as compared to normal myocardium. After a 10–30 minute delay, there is also more efficient egress of gadolinium from normal myocardium compared to infarcted or scarred tissue, further increasing the gradient of volume of distribution between normal and infarcted/fibrosed myocardium. This leads to greater signal intensity (bright signal) compared

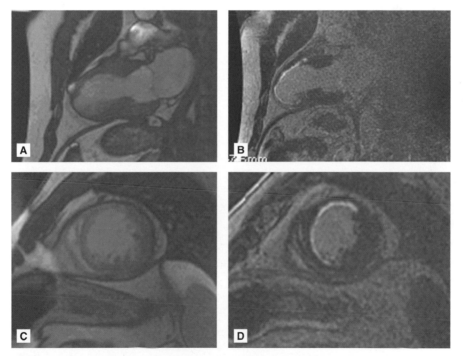

FIGURE 6.6   End-systolic gradient echo images (*A* and *C*) with corresponding delayed enhancement images (*B* and *D*) in a patient with previous myocardial infarction. There is thinned myocardium in the mid and distal anterior apex and distal inferior apex (*A*) as well as mid anterior and mid anteroseptal segments (*C*). On delayed enhancement imaging, there is subendocardial delayed enhancement in the mid and distal anterior and distal inferior segments (*B*). On short axis view (*D*), there is subendocardial delayed enhancement in the mid anteroseptum, mid inferoseptum, and mid inferior septum.

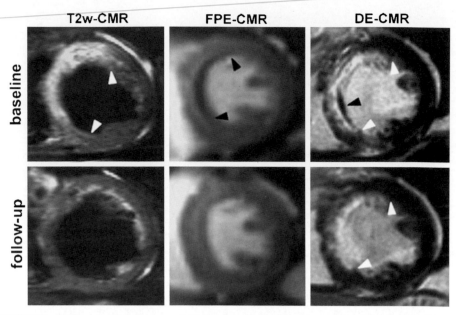

FIGURE 6.7 CMR evaluation of myocardial infarction. First column shows T2 weighted spin echo evaluation of the mid ventricle (short axis view). At baseline (*top row*), there is enhanced signal intensity in the anterior and anteroseptal segments compared to the rest of the myocardium, suggesting myocardial edema. On follow-up examination months later, there is now isointense signal in this region compared to the rest of the myocardium, signifying resolution of myocardial edema. Middle column shows first pass perfusion showing subendocardial signal loss in the same regions at baseline (*top*) that persists but to a lesser extent on follow-up (*bottom*). This shows reduced perfusion in these regions. Third column shows delayed enhancement showing both nontransmural as well as transmural delayed enhancement in the anterior, anteroseptum, and inferoseptum (*top, white arrows*). In the inferoseptum, there is a dark band in the subendocardium (*top, black arrow*) representing microvascular obstruction. On follow-up examination, the regions show delayed enhancement signifying myocardial scar and fibrosis.

Hombach V, Grebe O, Merkle N, et al. Sequelae of acute myocardial infarction regarding cardiac structure and function and their prognostic significance as assessed by magnetic resonance imaging. *European Heart Journal.* 2005; 26:549–557, by permission of the European Society of Cardiology.

to normal myocardium, a phenomenon called delayed enhancement. By using inversion recovery pulse prior to image acquisition to flip the magnetization of both normal and infarcted myocardium, one can further exploit the signal differences between the two regions. Because infarcted or scarred myocardium has higher volume of distribution of gadolinium, signal recovery occurs faster than in normal myocardium. If image acquisition is timed during the crossing of the normal myocardium's recovering signal at the null point (the inversion time), normal myocardium would appear dark while infarcted or scarred myocardium would appear bright (Figure 6.6 and 6.7).

Because of the high spatial resolution of MRI, subendocardial infarcts can now be detected. The amount of infarct or scar within a segment, assessed either by area or by transmural extent, determines the likelihood of functional recovery following revascularization or viability. Since the inverse relationship between the extent of delayed enhancement and functional recovery is a continuum, meaningful cutoff thresholds to dichotomize between viability and nonviability depend on clinically acceptable sensitivity and specificity. Thus, although <25% transmural extent of delayed enhancement best predicts post-revascularization recovery and >75% best predicts lack of recovery, CMR practitioners have used 50% transmural extent as a clinically useful threshold to guide them in determining viability of a myocardial segment. Other factors that may guide in the assessment include diastolic wall thickness with greater than 5.5 mm, which is indicative of myocardial viability and, as previously mentioned, biphasic response with dobutamine infusion signifying contractile reserve.

The amount of delayed enhancement following myocardial infarction has been shown to predict long-term survival.

Microvascular Obstruction

Unique to CMR, we now have the ability to detect microvascular obstruction following acute myocardial infarction and subsequent revascularization. Microvascular obstruction occurs when there is profound disruption of the capillary network as a result of ischemic insult such that blood flow is not established in the region following restoration of epicardial coronary flow. Microvascular obstruction appears as a perfusion defect on first pass gadolinium imaging and as a dark central area surrounded by regions of high signal intensity on delayed enhancement imaging (Figure 6.7). The lack of signal at the central core is caused by the inability of gadolinium to reach the area of profound microvascular disruption. The presence of microvascular obstruction is an independent predictor of mortality.

Acute versus Chronic Infarct

The ability of CMR to detect tissue contrast can be exploited to determine whether an area of infarct is acute or chronic. In both cases, inflammation and fibrosis within the myocardium will lead to delayed enhancement as a result of relative increased volume of distribution of gadolinium versus normal myocardium. It has been shown that within days, the amount of delayed enhancement is reduced as a result of reduced inflammation, with the remaining region of delayed enhancement representing infarcted region with scar and fibrosis. By using T2 weighted spin echo imaging, areas with relatively higher water content (such as inflamed myocardium from acute infarction) will appear to have higher signal intensity compared to normal myocardium (Figure 6.7). Chronic infarct associated with established scar and fibrosis, on the other hand, will appear isointense to normal myocardium on T2 weighted imaging. T2 weighted spin echo images in addition to delayed enhancement gradient echo images are useful in quantifying the extent of infarction and its relative age.

Ischemic versus Nonischemic Cardiomyopathy

Delayed enhancement is not, however, specific for ischemic heart disease. Areas of fibrosis or infiltration in the myocardium from nonischemic causes would show similar increased relative volume of distribution of gadolinium with bright signal. Delayed enhancement from ischemic heart disease follows coronary territory distribution, is either subendocardial or transmural, and is frequently associated with segmental wall motion abnormality. Nonischemic cardiomyopathy delayed enhancement distribution may not follow coronary territories and may be seen in the mid myocardium or epicardium (Figure 6.8). This difference in the pattern of delayed enhancement may be useful in the noninvasive evaluation of patients presenting with left ventricular dysfunction, especially in those at higher risk for invasive cardiac catheterization. It must be noted, however, that a small proportion of patients with nonischemic cardiomyopathy may present with a subendocardial or transmural delayed enhancement pattern similar to coronary artery disease.

FIGURE 6.8 Patterns of delayed enhancement. A. Coronary artery disease (CAD) subjects present with subendocardial or transmural delayed enhancement post-gadolinium that follows coronary artery territory distribution. This pattern is also seen 13% of dilated cardiomyopathy (DCMP) patients. B. Midmyocardial delayed enhancement such as shown in the septum (arrows) is a pattern seen in 28% of DCMP subjects but not CAD or normal subjects. C. Absence of delayed enhancement is seen in all normal subjects and 59% of DCMP patients. From McCrohon JA, Moon JCC, Prasad SK, et al. Differentiation of heart failure related to dilated cardiomyopathy and coronary artery disease using gadolinium-enhanced cardiovascular magnetic resonance. *Circulation.* 2003; 108:54–59.

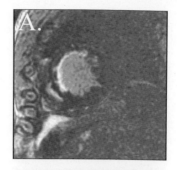

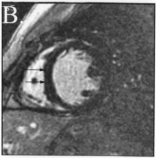

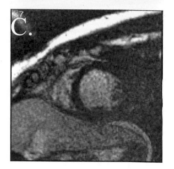

Sequelae and Complications of Myocardial Infarction

The ability of CMR to perform cardiac imaging using unlimited planes with high spatial resolution, as well as the ability to perform tissue contrast imaging, are useful in the assessment of complications of myocardial infarction.

Left Ventricular Aneurysms and Pseudoaneurysms

Left ventricular aneurysms and pseudoaneurysms can be assessed with static black blood/spin echo images or with the dynamic cine bright blood/gradient echo technique. Both techniques allow for evaluation of the presence of wall thinning and contour abnormalities, determination of their location and morphology, and assessment for potential complication of pericardial effusion associated with aneurysm/pseudoaneurysm rupture. Dynamic bright blood imaging not only demonstrates the regional wall dyskinesia and outpouching during systole, but it can also help identify the presence of mural thrombus within the aneurysm sac.

True left ventricular aneurysms are characterized by focal wall thinning extending from the endocardium to the pericardium (Figure 6.9). They tend to have large ostia in comparison to the internal diameter of the sac. Most true aneurysms are located along the anterolateral and apical walls of the left ventricle.

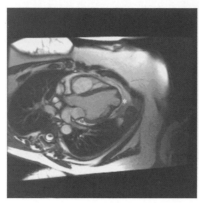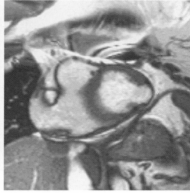

FIGURE 6.9 Focal aneurysm in the distal inferolateral segment. Steady-state free precession gradient echo at end-systole demonstrates focal outpouching of the ventricle. The ostial width is comparable in size to the width of the sac body, suggesting that this is a focal post-infarct true aneurysm.

A pseudoaneurysm of the left ventricle is usually secondary to a localized but contained rupture of the ventricle into the pericardial space. It is termed a pseudoaneurysm as it is not composed of all three layers of the heart; rather, a layer of pericardium composes the wall. Pseudoaneurysms tend to have ostia that are considerably smaller than the internal diameter of the aneurysm sac itself. Additionally, pseudoaneurysms caused by myocardial infarcts are usually located along the posterolateral and diaphragmatic walls of the left ventricle.

The differentiation between true aneurysm and pseudoaneurysm is critical, as the latter is associated with increased mortality and likelihood of rupture. Therefore, the decision for urgent surgical intervention often underlies the distinction between the two. However, the only accurate way to distinguish true from false left ventricular aneurysm is with histologic analysis of the aneurysm wall. Clinically, the ratio of ostium diameter to the sac diameter is frequently used to differentiate the two. The presence of pericardial effusion, although a non-specific finding, may also be a more ominous sign if it results from bleeding into the pericardial space. The disruption of the epicardial fat layer has been cited as a sign of pseudoaneurysm, but spatial resolution limitations make this finding very difficult to assess.

Left Ventricular Thrombus

Intracardiac thrombus can occur in any area demonstrating low or slow blood flow. In the setting of ischemic heart disease, slow flow is usually seen within true or false ventricular aneurysms within a severely dysfunctional left ventricle, or within an enlarged left atrial chamber from mitral valvular disease. Thrombus may also be seen in the area adjacent to myocardial infarcts, even in the absence of aneurysm. Recognizing intracardiac thrombus is important for initiation of anticoagulation to decrease risk of systemic embolization. Transthoracic echocardiography is the usual first-line imaging modality to evaluate intracardiac thrombus. Mural thrombi may, however, be difficult to visualize with echo, possibly because of the size or location of the thrombus or similar acoustic characteristics with myocardium. Cardiac magnetic resonance imaging has been shown to be useful in identifying and characterizing intracardiac thrombus. Although spin echo sequences may demonstrate the thrombus, slow flow in the region or in-plane flow may result in signal intensity within the ventricular cavity that is difficult to distinguish from thrombus. Gradient echo cine techniques, especially steady-state free precession, demonstrate good tissue contrast between blood pool and myocardium with high spatial resolution, and are therefore useful for demonstrating

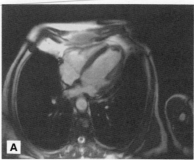 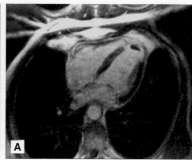

FIGURE 6.10 Apical thrombus. (*A*) Steady-state free precession gradient echo sequence showing a dark signal intensity mass in the apex between the myocardium and the bright blood pool. (*B*) Delayed enhancement imaging reveals the contrast between the dark signal intensity thrombus between the bright blood pool signal and the bright myocardial signal as a result of transmural delayed enhancement in the apex (apical infarct).

intracardiac thrombus, which would appear as dark areas within the ventricular cavity adjacent to endocardium (Figure 6.10). In addition, first pass perfusion as well as delayed enhancement imaging following gadolinium administration allow for identification of the thrombus. Thrombus does not take up gadolinium and will appear dark in contrast to the bright blood pool signal and the underlying bright delayed enhancement of the infarcted myocardium. In a comparative study, CMR had higher sensitivity and specificity for detecting intracardiac thrombus in coronary artery disease as compared to both transthoracic and transesophageal echocardiography.[12]

Ventricular Septal Defect

Ventricular septal defects (VSD) caused by infarction and subsequent disruption of the ventricular septum can be identified using spin echo as well as gradient echo imaging. The ability to use unlimited imaging planes is an advantage of CMR in delineating the extent and location of VSD. In the setting of acute infarction, the presence of this mechanical complication is most often a surgical indication for repair. The amount of shunting, therefore, is less an issue for surgical decision making than it is in adult congenital ventricular septal defects, owing to a different natural course. Shunts can be quantified by CMR by accurately measuring the stroke volume of the left and right ventricles, and determining the ratio of pulmonic flow to aortic flow. In the absence of significant atrioventricular valve regurgitation, stroke volume can be assessed either by using phase contrast cine just above the aortic and pulmonic valves to quantify flow, or by using the difference between end-diastolic and end-systolic volumes of the left and right ventricles. Cine phase contrast pulse sequence is used to measure velocity and flow. With this technique, moving spins accrue a net phase proportional to velocity. Both phase and magnitude images are generated. Phase images contain velocity data, while magnitude images provide anatomic definition. By accumulating data involving a specified region of interest (a vessel or flow jet), time-velocity and time-flow curves can be generated from which flow can be quantified.

Ischemic Mitral Regurgitation

Ischemia of the papillary muscle may lead to rupture of the muscle head or chordal structures, leading to mitral regurgitation. Often this mechanical complication is associated with profound heart failure and necessitates urgent surgical intervention. In addition, adverse chronic ventricular remodeling from myocardial infarction may lead to apical tethering, poor coaptation of mitral leaflets, and mitral regurgitation. Echocardiography is the first-line tool in the assessment of valvular disease. With poor acoustic windows and in conjunction with other tests such as delayed enhancement imaging, CMR can be used to assess the extent and mechanism of mitral regurgitation. The unlimited imaging planes will allow full evaluation of the mitral apparatus that will be helpful in determining the mechanism of regurgitation. Furthermore, accurate evaluation of ventricular volumes, function, and mass will be useful in serial follow-up to assess the morphologic effects of mitral regurgitation. Black blood/spin echo sequences can be used to assess valvular leaflet morphology. However, dynamic cine bright blood/gradient echo images are usually used as this sequence can examine leaflet morphology as well as valvular motion and dysfunction, and can be used to evaluate the presence of dark flow jets or signal voids against the background of a bright blood pool. With dynamic imaging, evaluation of valvular motion/dysfunction, including assessment of annular enlargement, leaflet prolapse, or leaflet restriction, can be performed. Qualitative assessment of the degree of mitral regurgitation is done by evaluating the degree of dark signal intensity in the atrial region during systole using a gradient echo pulse sequence. Dark jets signify areas of fast or turbulent flow and are caused by a phenomenon referred to as intravoxel dephasing. Semiquantitative assessment of valvular dysfunction can be obtained by measuring the area, extent, and duration of signal void on the bright blood sequences. Quantification of the degree of mitral regurgitation is done by measuring the regurgitant volume using phase contrast imaging through the mitral valve or, alternatively, calculating the difference between left ventricular stroke volume (end-diastolic minus end-systolic volume by cine) and aortic forward flow using phase contrast cine across the aortic valve.

Summary

Cardiac magnetic resonance imaging offers true comprehensive evaluation of coronary artery disease, including evaluation of structure, function, perfusion and ischemia, coronary stenosis, infarction, myocardial viability, valvular dysfunction, and mechanical complications. Its advantages include lack of ionizing radiation, safety, high spatial resolution, unlimited imaging planes, good image quality in patients with poor acoustic windows or who are prone to radiotracer attenuation, and excellent tissue contrast. Its disadvantages include relatively long acquisition time (typically 45–60 minutes), inability to image patients with ferromagnetic materials or claustrophobia, lack of true real-time imaging capability and dependence on good cardiac gating, relative cost, and availability. With constant improvement in both software and hardware, it is anticipated that most of these issues will be addressed. Among all the modalities available, cardiac MRI offers the greatest potential for a "one stop shop" noninvasive evaluation of coronary artery disease.

REFERENCES

1. Grothues F, Smith GC, Moon JC, et al. Comparison of interstudy reproducibility of cardiovascular magnetic resonance with two-dimensional echocardiography in normal subjects and in patients with heart failure or left ventricular hypertrophy. *Am J Cardiol.* 2002; 90:29–34.
2. Lorenz CH, Walker ES, Morgan VL, et al. Normal human right and left ventricular mass, systolic function, and gender differences by cine magnetic resonance imaging. *J Cardiovasc Magn Reson.* 1999; 1:7–21.
3. Klem I, Heitner J, Shah D, et al. Improved detection of coronary atery disease by stress perfusion cardiovascular magnetic resonance with the use of delayed enhancement infarct imaging. *JACC.* 2006; 47:1630–1638.
4. Positano V, Pingitore A, Scattini B, et al. Myocardial perfusion by first pass contrast magnetic resonance: a robust method for quantitative regional assessment of perfusion reserve index. *Heart.* 2006; 92(5):689–690.
5. Sakuma H, Suzawa N, Ichikawa Y, et al. Diagnostic Accuracy of Stress First-Pass Contrast-Enhanced Myocardial Perfusion MRI Compared with Stress Myocardial Perfusion Scintigraphy. *Am J Roentgenol.* 2005; 185(1):95–102.
6. Wolff S, Schwitter J, Coulden R, et al. Myocardial first-pass perfusion magnetic resonance imaging: A multicenter dose-ranging study. *Circulation.* 2004; 110:732–737.
7. Nagel E, Klein C, Paetsch I, et al. Magnetic Resonance Perfusion Measurements for the Noninvasive Detection of Coronary Artery Disease. *Circulation.* 2003; 108(4):432–437.

8. Ishida N, Sakuma H, Motoyasu M, et al. Noninfarcted myocardium: correlation between dynamic first-pass contrast-enhanced myocardial MR imaging and quantitative coronary angiography. *Radiology*. 2003; 229(1):209–216.

9. Schwitter J, Nanz D, Kneifel S, et al. Assessment of Myocardial Perfusion in Coronary Artery Disease by Magnetic Resonance: A Comparison With Positron Emission Tomography and Coronary Angiography. *Circulation*. 2001; 103(18):2230–2235.

10. Nagel E, Lehmkuhl HB, Bocksch W, et al. Noninvasive diagnosis of ischemia-induced wall motion abnormalities with the use of high-dose dobutamine stress MRI: comparison with dobutamine stress echocardiography. *Circulation*. 1999; 99(6):763–770.

11. Kim WY, Danias PG, Stuber M, et al. Coronary magnetic resonance angiography for the detection of coronary stenoses. *N Engl J Med*. 2001; 345:1863–1869.

12. Srichai MB, Junor C, Rodriguez LL, et al. Clinical, imaging, and pathological characteristics of left ventricular thrombus: A comparison of contrast-enhanced magnetic resonance imaging, transthoracic echocardiography, and transesophageal echocardiography with surgical or pathological validation. *Am Heart J*. 2006; 152:75–84.

Abbara S, Miller SW. Pericardial and myocardial disease. In: Miller SW, ed. *The Requisites: Cardiac Imaging*. 2nd ed. Philadelphia: Elsevier Mosby; 2005:245–283.

Abdel-Aty H, Zarosek A, Schulz-Menger J, et al. Delayed enhancement and T2-weighted cardiovascular magnetic resonance imaging differentiate acute from chronic myocardial infarction. *Circulation*. 2004; 109:2411–2416.

Baer F, Theissen P, Schneider C, et al. Dobutamine magnetic resonance imaging predicts contractile recovery of chronically dysfunctional myocardium after successful revascularization. *J Am Coll Cardiol*. 1998; 31:1040–1048.

Beek A, Kuhl H, Bondarenko O, et al. Delayed contrast-enhanced magnetic resonance imaging for the prediction of regional functional improvement after acute myocardial infarction. *J Am Coll Cardiol*. 2003; 42:895–901.

Bottini P, Carr A, Prisant L, et al. Magnetic resonance imaging compared to echocardiography to assess left ventricular mass in the hypertensive patient. *Am J Hypertens*. 1995; 8:221–228.

Boxt L. Cardiac magnetic resonance imaging. In: Miller SW, ed. *The Requisites: Cardiac Imaging*. 2nd ed. Philadelphia: Elsevier Mosby; 2005:88–131.

Cecil M, Kosinski A, Jones M, et al. The importance of work-up (verification) bias correction in assessing the accuracy of SPECT Thallium-201 testing for the diagnosis of coronary artery disease. *J Clin. Epidemiol*. 1996; 49:735–742.

Cerqueira M, Weissman N, Dilsizian V, et al. Standardized myocardial segmentation and nomenclature for tomographic imaging of the heart: A statement for healthcare professionals from the cardiac imaging committee of the council on clinical cardiology of the American Heart Association. *J Nucl Cardiol*. 200; 9:240–245.

Choi K, Kim R, Gubernikoff G, et al. Transmural extent of acute myocardial infarction predicts long-term improvement in contractile function. *Circulation*. 2001; 104:1101–1107.

Cowper SE. Nephrogenic Fibrosing Dermopathy [NFD/NSF Website]. 2001–2007. Available at http://www.icnfdr.org. Accessed 04/2007.

Glockner J, Johnston D, and McGee K. Evaluation of cardiac valvular disease with MR imaging: Qualitative and quantitative techniques. *RadioGraphics*. 2003; 23:9.

Gould T. How MRI works. http://www.howstuffworks.com/mri.htm (Apr. 2007).

Higgins C. Magnetic resonance imaging of ischemic heart disease. In: Webb WR, Higgins C, eds. *Thoracic Imaging: Pulmonary and Cardiovascular Radiology*. Philadelphia: Lippincott Williams & Wilkins; 2005:774–779.

Higgins C, Krombach G. Cardiac and paracardiac masses. In: Webb WR, Higgins C, eds. *Thoracic Imaging: Pulmonary and Cardiovascular Radiology*. Philadelphia: Lippincott Williams & Wilkins; 2005:735–750.

Kaandorp TA, Lamb HJ, van der Wall EE, et al. Cardiovascular MR to assess myocardial viability in chronic ischemic LV dysfunction. *Heart*. 2005; 91:1359–1365.

Kim RJ, Wu E, Rafael A, et al. The use of contrast-enhanced magnetic resonance imaging to identify reversible myocardial dysfunction. *N Engl J Med*. 2000; 343:1445–1453.

Klein C, Nekolla S, Bengel F, et al. Assessment of myocardial viability with contrast-enhanced magnetic resonance imaging: Comparison with positron emission tomography. *Circulation*. 2002; 105:162–167.

Klepac S, Samett E. (Last updated 1/24/2007) Cardiac MRI—Technical aspects primer. http://www.emedicine.com/radio/topic866.htm (Apr 2007)

Kwong RY, Chan AK, Brown KA, et al. Impact of unrecognized myocardial scar detected by cardiac magnetic resonance imaging on event-free survival in patients presenting with signs and symptoms of coronary artery disease. *Circulation*. 2006; 113:2733–2743.

Lima D, Desai M. Cardiovascular magnetic resonance imaging: Current and emerging applications. *J Am Coll Cardiol*. 2004; 44:1164–1171.

Micromedex, Facts & Comparisons, and Multum (2007) http://www.drugs.com/pro/Adenosine.html (Apr. 2007).

Miller T, Hedge D, Christian T, et al. Effects of adjustment for referral bias on the sensitivity and specificity of single photon emission computed tomography for the diagnosis of coronary artery disease. *Am J Med*. 2002; 112:290–297.

Mollet N, Dymarkowski S, Volders W, et al. Visualization of ventricular thrombi with contrast-enhanced magnetic resonance imaging in patients with ischemic heart disease. *Circulation*. 2002; 106:2873–2876.

Nagel E, Lehmkuhl H, Bocksch W, et al. Noninvasive diagnosis of ischemia-induced wall motion abnormalities with use of high-dose dobutamine stress MRI: Comparison with dobutamine stress echocardiography. *Circulation*. 1999; 99:763–770.

Pennell D. Cardiovascular magnetic resonance and the role of Adenosine pharmacologic stress. *Am J Cardiol*. 2004; 94(suppl):26D–32D.

Pohost G, Hung L, and Doyle M. Clinical use of cardiovascular magnetic resonance. *Circulation*. 2003; 108:647–653

Post JC, van Rossum AC, Bronzwaer JGF, et al. Magnetic resonance angiography of anomalous coronary arteries: A new gold standard for delineating the proximal course? *Circulation*. 1995; 92:3163–3171.

Sadowski E, Bennett L, Chan M, et al. Nephrogenic systemic fibrosis: Risk factors and incidence estimation. *Radiology*. 2007; 243:148–157.

Schuijf JD, Shaw LJ, Wijns W, et al. Cardiac imaging in coronary artery disease: Differing modalities. *Heart*. 2005; 91:1110–1117.

Smart S, Sawada S, Ryan T, et al. Low-dose dobutamine echocardiography detects reversible dysfunction after thrombolytic therapy of acute myocardial infarction. *Circulation*. 1993; 88:405–415.

Stork A, Muellerleile K, Bansmann P, et al. Value of T2-weighted, first-pass and delayed enhancement, and cine CMR to differentiate between acute and chronic myocardial infarction. *Eur Radiol*. 2007; 17:610–617.

Tan R, Chen K. Coronary artery disease: Comprehensive evaluation by cardiovascular magnetic resonance imaging. *Ann Acad Med*. 2004; 33:437–443.

Taylor A, Al-Saadi N, Abdel-Aty H, et al. Detection of acutely impaired microvascular reperfusion after infarct angioplasty with magnetic resonance imaging. *Circulation*. 2004; 109:2080–2085.

Underwood SR, Anagnostopoulos C, Cerqueira M, et al. Myocardial perfusion scintigraphy: The evidence. *Eur J Nucl Med Mol Imag*. 2004; 31:261–291.

Wagner S, Auffermann W, Buser P, et al. Diagnostic accuracy and estimation of the severity of valvular regurgitation from the signal void on cine magnetic resonance images. *Am Heart J*. 1989; 118:760–767.

Wagner A, Mahrholdt H, Holly TA, et al. Contrast-enhanced MRI and routine single photon emission computed tomography (SPECT) perfusion imaging for detection of subendocardial myocardial infarcts: An imaging study. *Lancet*. 2003; 361:274–379.

Wicky S, Miller SW. Ischemic heart disease. In: Miller SW, ed. *The Requisites: Cardiac Imaging*. 2ne ed. Philadelphia: Elsevier Mosby; 2005:202–283.

Wu KC, Zerhouni EA, Judd RM, et al. Prognostic significance of microvascular obstruction by magnetic resonance imaging in patients with acute myocardial infarction. *Circulation*. 1998; 97:765–772.

Risk Stratification Using Inflammatory Markers and Other Risk Factors in Nuclear Imaging

Risk Factors and Stratification in Chronic CAD

Research into risk factors for coronary artery disease (CAD) has continued to refine the stratification of patients with potential and diagnosed CAD.[1] Innumerable reports have used myocardial perfusion imaging (MPI) to classify patient characteristics to better assess an individual's risk for CAD. However, more recently, intense research has focused on a vast array of inflammatory markers that can potentially be used in conjunction with currently available clinical and radiologic findings. Despite the advances in the identification of inflammatory markers and their role in CAD, the current guidelines for prevention, detection, and evaluation of patients at risk for CAD do not recommend their routine use.[2]

Potential Use of Inflammatory Markers[3,4]

The ideal characteristics of a marker for coronary artery disease are as follows: First, a marker has to be identified as having a potential relation with endothelial damage or other inflammatory processes associated with CAD.[5] Second, it should be inexpensive, easy to standardize, have clear cut-off points, and have a high sensitivity. Third, it should stand up to the scrutiny of population-based trials where its presence (or absence) has independent predictive value (Figure 7.1).[6] Although some consider hs-CRP to be an exception, there is currently no marker available that fulfills all the above characteristics. However, algorithms have been developed that incorporate some of these markers to add to the predictive value of other forms of risk stratification.[7]

C-Reactive Protein[8,9]

C-reactive protein (CRP) is a well-established acute phase reactant that has recently been identified as a major cardiovascular risk factor by using higher sensitivity assays (hs-CRP). It is expressed in smooth muscle cells within diseased arteries and has been found to play a role in atherogenesis and plaque vulnerability.[10] It has prognostic value during acute ischemic events and in patients with established CAD. However, its most relevant use is in the setting of primary prevention. Several major studies have confirmed that it has an additive value to the Framingham risk score and to other markers such as low-density lipoprotein (LDL) cholesterol (Figure 7.2),[11] though the degree to which it is predictive of CAD is still under discussion.[12]

Homocysteine

Increased concentration of homocysteine may result in vascular changes, including impairment of endothelial function, enhanced thrombogenesis, and smooth muscle cell proliferation.[13] Also, elevated homocysteine levels have been correlated with CAD risk in some

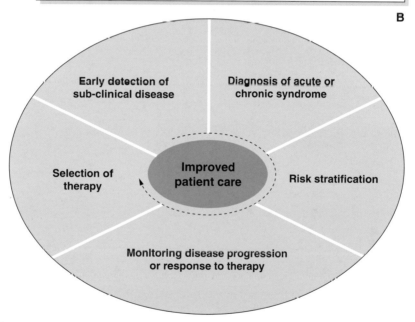

1) Can the clinician measure the biomarker?   **A**

  a) Accurate and reproducible analytical method(s)
  b) Pre-analytical issues (including stability) evaluated and manageable
  c) Assay is accessible
  d) Available assays provide high throughput and rapid turnaround
  e) Reasonable cost

2) Does the biomarker add new information?

  a) Strong and consistent association between the biomarker and the
     outcome or disease of interest in multiple studies
  b) Information adds to or improves upon existing tests
  c) Decision-limits are validated in more than one study
  d) Evaluation includes the data from community-based populations

3) Will the biomarker help the clinician to manage patients?

  a) Superior performance to existing diagnostic tests, or
  b) Evidence that associated risk is modifiable with specific therapy, or
  c) Evidence that biomarker-guided triage or monitoring enhances care
  d) Consider each of multiple potential uses (See Panel B)

                                                                                     B

Early detection of sub-clinical disease

Diagnosis of acute or chronic syndrome

Selection of therapy

Improved patient care

Risk stratification

Monitoring disease progression or response to therapy

FIGURE 7.1   (*A*) Criteria for assessment of novel cardiovascular biomarkers for clinical use. (*B*) Clinical applications of cardiovascular biomarkers.
From Morrow DA, de Lemos JA. Benchmarks for the assessment of novel cardiovascular biomarkers. *Circulation.* 2007; 115:949 952.

case-control studies, but the data is not as clear in prospective studies.[14] Although it has also been shown that folic acid supplementation reduces levels of homocysteine, its use has not been shown to decrease the risk of cardiovascular disease. In most cases the measurement of homocysteine levels is not indicated in the evaluation or risk stratification of patients with suspected or known CAD.

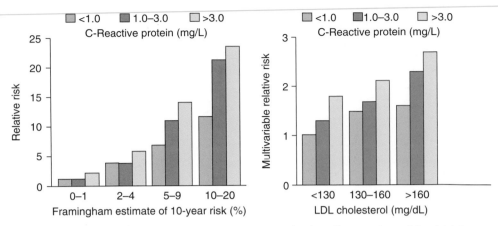

FIGURE 7.2   Additive value of high-sensitivity C-reactive protein after adjustment for traditional risk factors. Data are shown across all levels of low-density lipoprotein (LDL) cholesterol (*right*) and across all levels of calculated Framingham risk (*left*).
Adapted from Ridker PM, Rifai N, Rose L, Buring JE, Cook NR. Comparison of C-reactive protein and low-density lipoprotein cholesterol levels in the prediction of fist cardiovascular events. *N Engl J Med.* 2002; 347:1557–1565.

Erythrocyte Sedimentation Rate[15]

Erythrocyte sedimentation rate (ESR) is a very sensitive marker of inflammation that has been extensively studied in various diseases. A meta-analysis of several population-based studies using ESR concluded that there was mildly relevant—but statistically significant—use for it as a marker for CAD. Based on these studies, the use of ESR is not advocated in further classifying patients for potential CAD.

Others
Fibrinogen[16]
Fibrinogen is very relevant in the clot formation process. It is also an acute phase reactant that has been studied as a possible marker for CAD. In several studies it was demonstrated to have predictive value. However, it has not been accepted into routine clinical practice because of the difficultly in standardization.

Interleukin-6[17]
Interleukin-6 (IL-6) is a powerful inducer of the hepatic acute phase response and is the primary determinant for C-reactive protein production. IL-6 decreases lipoprotein lipase (LPL) activity in plasma, which increases macrophage uptake of lipids. Macrophage foam cells and smooth muscle cells (SMC) express IL-6, suggesting a role for this cytokine along with interleukin-1 (IL-1) and tumor necrosis factor-α (TNF-α) in the progression of atherosclerosis.[18] In prospective studies it has been shown to be mildly predictive of future coronary events in apparently healthy populations,[19,20] though its prognostic value over other markers has not been clearly established because of its high variability.

Lipoprotein Associated Phospholipase A2
Lipoprotein associated phospholipase A2 (Lp-PLA2) is secreted by macrophages, T-cells, and mast cells and is transported through the body mostly via LDL. Over-expression of Lp-PLA2 has been found in different populations to both increase and decrease risk for CAD, and animal studies have suggested that it is mostly a pro-atherogenic protein. Research is still ongoing and most agree that additional data are needed to elucidate its role.

Plasminogen Activator Inhibitor-1[21,22]

Plasminogen activator inhibitor-1 (PAI-1) has been shown to exert a pro-atherothrombotic effect on endothelial cells. There are epidemiological studies that PAI-1 excess may contribute to the development of ischemic cardiovascular disease. In vivo administration of antibodies against PAI-1 has been proven effective in preventing development of thrombus in transgenic mice expressing human PAI-1 develop coronary arterial thrombosis.[23] To date, PAI-1 has not been used as a marker for stable coronary artery disease, but preliminary data indicates that it may be useful at the time surrounding an acute coronary event as plasma PAI-1 activity has been noted to be increased in MI survivors that later develop recurrent MI.

Imaging Findings

Beyond the finding of ischemia during MPI there are other less commonly used but potentially useful indicators of CAD, such as ejection fraction and ischemic dilatation. These findings are particularly applicable in high and medium risk patients that have mild to moderate ischemia.

Left Ventricular Ejection Fraction

It is well established that ejection fraction (EF) is inversely related with cardiac mortality. With the assistance of currently available software, it is now commonplace to evaluate ejection fraction along with perfusion during a standard MPI. This "added" information should be considered in the overall cardiac evaluation, as post-stress EF seems to be closely related to the likelihood of cardiac death (Figure 7.3).[24]

Number of Reversible Defects

The presence of increasing amounts of ischemia after treadmill stress testing has been shown to correlate with higher likelihood of nonfatal myocardial infarction.[25] The relation holds up in patients with low, intermediate, and high-risk results post exercise.[26]

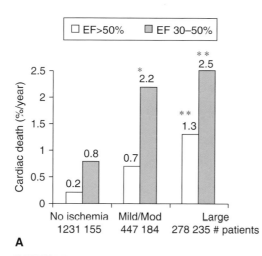
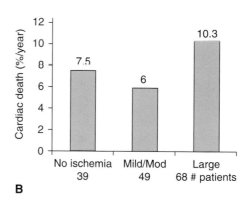

FIGURE 7.3 Cardiac death rate as a function of amount of ischemia in patients with ejection fraction (EF) >50% and EF between 30% and 50% (*A*) and in patients with EF <30% (*B*). Mod, moderate. *$p < 0.05$ vs. EF >50% in same perfusion category. **$p < 0.005$ compared with no ischemia and same EF category. Sharir T, Germano G, Kang X, et al. Prediction of myocardial infarction versus cardiac death by gated myocardial perfusion SPECT: Risk stratification by the amount of stress-induced ischemia and the poststress ejection fraction. *J Nucl Med. 2001*; 42:831–837, with permission.

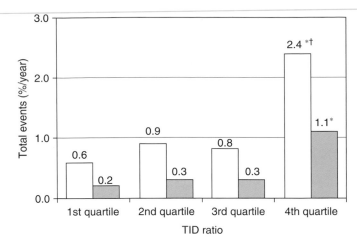

FIGURE 7.4 Annual rates of first future cardiac events (total events) and hard events in patients with normal myocardial perfusion single photon emission computed tomography distributed by quartiles of transient ischemic dilation (TID) ratio. *$p < 0.001$ across the groups; †$p = 0.006$ for highest quartile versus all others. Open bars = total events; solid bars = hard events.

Reprinted from Abidov A, Baxx J, Hayes SW, et al. Transient ischemic dilaton ratio of the left ventricle is a significant predictor of future cardiac events in patients with otherwise normal myocardial perfusion SPECT. *J Am Coll Cardiol.* 2003; 42:1818–1825, with permission from Elsevier.

Other Nuclear Findings

An increased amount of Tl-201 lung uptake and transient ischemic dilation (TID > 1.20) are both associated with increased risk of cardiac morbidity and mortality and have additive value to other clinical findings such as diabetes, angina, and advanced age (Figure 7.4).[27]

Dyspnea[28] and Character of Chest Pain[29]

The presence of anginal symptoms before and during stress testing is prognostic of future events and increases the likelihood of positive MPI. A review of over 20,000 patients at a single center reported that the anginal symptoms per se, and more specifically typical anginal symptoms, slightly increased the risk for future cardiac events after stress testing. This same trial also showed that the presence of dyspnea prior to stress testing resulted in a dramatically worse outcome than any other chest pain symptom (Figure 7.5).

Computerized Tomography

It has been found that the amount of calcification in the coronary arteries roughly correlates with the severity of the underlying atherosclerotic burden. Coronary artery scanning with computed tomography angiogram (CTA) has been found to be a viable method for identifying coronary obstruction and quantifying the degree of calcification. Even though some clarification of the data is still needed, several studies[30] have used calcium scoring with CTA to reclassify patient risk for acute coronary events with similar—or greater—accuracy than traditional risk factor analysis. The currently used scoring is described in Agatston U as 0–100 being low, 100–400 moderate, and >400 as high risk,[31] but these cut-offs have not been universally accepted and adjustments can be made to take into account the age and sex of individual patients.[32]

A Patients with no known history of coronary artery disease

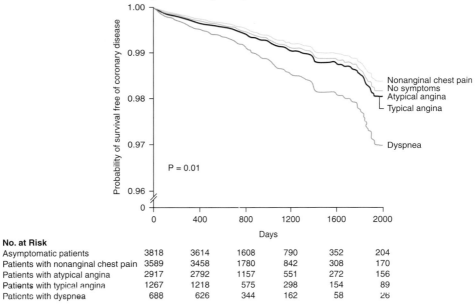

No. at Risk					
Asymptomatic patients	3818	3614	1608	790	352	204
Patients with nonanginal chest pain	3589	3458	1780	842	308	170
Patients with atypical angina	2917	2792	1157	551	272	156
Patients with typical angina	1267	1218	575	298	154	89
Patients with dyspnea	688	626	344	162	58	26

B Patients with a known history of coronary artery disease

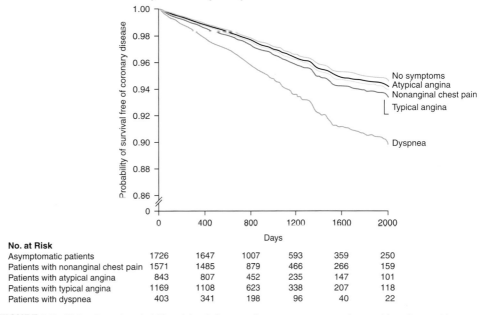

No. at Risk					
Asymptomatic patients	1726	1647	1007	593	359	250
Patients with nonanginal chest pain	1571	1485	879	466	266	159
Patients with atypical angina	843	807	452	235	147	101
Patients with typical angina	1169	1108	623	338	207	118
Patients with dyspnea	403	341	198	96	40	22

FIGURE 7.5 Risk-adjusted probability of death from cardiac causes among patients with no known history of coronary artery disease (*A*) and patients with a known history of coronary artery disease (*B*), according to the symptoms at presentation.
Abidov A, Rozanski A, Hachamovitch R, et al. Prognostic Significance of Dyspnea in Patients Referred for Cardiac Stress Testing http://content.nejm.org/cgi/content/short/ 353/18/1889. *N Engl J Med.* 2005; 353:1889–1898, Nov 3, 2005, with permission.

In Summary

The goal of risk stratification in patients with known or suspected coronary artery disease has been greatly elucidated. The advances in primary prevention of CAD have focused mainly on traditional risk factors, smoking, obesity, and hypertension. There have been aggressive public health campaigns for its early identification and modification with improved results. Basic research has identified several inflammatory molecules involved in the pathogenesis of CAD and a few of them have made their way to the clinical arena. Furthermore, in combination with nuclear imaging these have provided enhanced predictive capabilities. However, the major limitation is the identification of vulnerable coronary plaques in patients who are asymptomatic and at a high risk for an acute coronary event.

Risk Stratification for Acute CAD

Background of Plaque Rupture[33]

The rupture of an unstable plaque in the coronary artery precedes the vast majority of acute myocardial infarctions. The pathology of an unstable plaque has been well documented and has classically been described as having a substantial amount of lipids, surrounded by a thin fibrous cap and very few smooth muscle cells. Because these lesions are usually non-obstructive they rarely occlude the vessel wall to a degree that can be detected by MPI prior to rupture.[34] This presents a significant gap in the capacity to elucidate and diagnose preemptively the presence of an unstable plaque prior to rupture.

Lipid Content

High lipid-content-to-fibrous-cap ratio is commonly seen in unstable plaques.[35] The cholesterol inside the lipid core has been described as being in a liquid state with some amount of crystallization. Formerly, these crystals had been described as inert, but the latest research has found that these crystals are capable of disrupting the fibrous cap and potentially initiating the baneful cascade that leads to acute plaque rupture and myocardial damage (Figure 7.6).[36]

As of now there are several imaging techniques available in academic centers such as magnetic resonance imaging, intravascular spectroscopy, and high resolution contrast tomography, that can accurately distinguish a high lipid content plaque from a low lipid/high fibrous cap plaque or a liquid lipid core from a crystallized lipid core, but unfortunately none of these techniques have been evaluated in the general population.

Cell-Mediated Processes[37]

Plaque rupture causes a cascade of cell-mediated events that cause thrombus formation, local and downstream inflammation, and subsequently complete occlusion of the coronary artery lumen. These processes include sometimes contradictory effects, as in T-cell production of interferon gamma that inhibits smooth muscle cell collagen synthesis and degranulation of platelets that increase collagen synthesis via tissue growth factor-β.

T-lymphocytes not only exert their plaque weakening effects via gamma interferon, they also signal via direct mechanisms for the activation of macrophages. Macrophages, activated by this and other signals such as oxidized lipoproteins, release metalloproteinases and elastolytic enzymes that promote matrix catabolism. This combination of decreased collagen synthesis and increased collagen degradation is at least partially to blame for the vulnerable characteristics of the unstable plaque.[38] The accumulation of apoptotic macrophages and smooth muscle cells inside the cholesterol-laden plaque generate particulate tissue factor and other inflammatory proteins that may also play a role in the subsequent plaque rupture.[39]

The creation of a large thrombus at the site of plaque rupture is an ominous event that is usually followed by a clinically evident injury to the myocardium. Small thrombi, on the

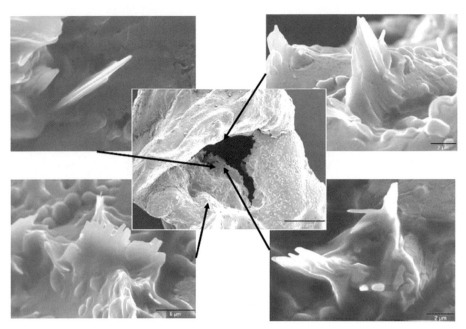

FIGURE 7.6   Scanning electron micrographs (SEM) of human left anterior descending coronary artery following plaque rupture in a 35-year-old male. SEM at low magnification of the whole artery (*middle image*) was obtained just below the rupture site. At higher magnification, pointed tipped cholesterol crystals are seen penetrating the intimal surface, causing major disruption of the endothelium at various sites (*arrows*). SEM preparation avoided ethanol in the dehydration process to prevent crystals from dissolving.
Abela GS, Aziz K. Cholesterol crystals rupture biological membranes and human plaques during acute cardiovascular events: A novel insight into plaque rupture by scanning electron microscopy. *Scanning.* 2006; 28:1–10, with permission.

other hand, have been found at the site of plaque rupture in non-ischemic hearts. It is not yet clear what events precede the formation of an obstructive thrombus, but histologically both leukocytes and platelets have been found to adhere to themselves and different areas of the ruptured plaque.

Identification of Vulnerable Plaque

There are very few, if any, clinically useful ways of identifying vulnerable plaques. As noted above, nuclear imaging techniques and associated biomarkers are mostly useful in identifying stable, advanced plaques that usually do not cause acute coronary events. A very similar statement can also be made with regard to cardiac catheterization.[40] CT scanning of the coronary vasculature with high resolution images may be useful in the near future for identifying vulnerable plaques, but with currently available technology it is, at best, only able to compare with coronary angiography in its capacity to detect obstruction in the coronary vasculature.[41] Angioscopy has been shown to be useful in detecting potentially unstable plaques based on yellow color implying a high lipid-content-to-fibrous-cap ratio. However, this is an invasive procedure that has not gained wide acceptance.[42] A novel technology that employs integrated backscanner intravascular ultrasound has recently been shown to be able to quantify the amount of cholesterol inside non-obstructive plaques in-vivo. Researchers have also shown that patients with metabolic syndrome have increased lipid content and may be subject to a higher risk of plaque rupture.[43]

FIGURE 7.7 Correlation between fluorodeoxyglucose (FDG) uptake and macrophage density in rabbit aortic specimens. There was a significant correlation between FDG activity and macrophage density ($r = 0.79$, $p < 0.001$). Reprinted from Tawakol A, Migrino RQ, Hoffmann U, et al. Noninvasive in vivo measurement of vascular inflammation with F-18 fluorodeoxyglucose positron emission tomography. *J Nucl Cardiol.* 2005: 12:294–301, with permission from Elsevier.

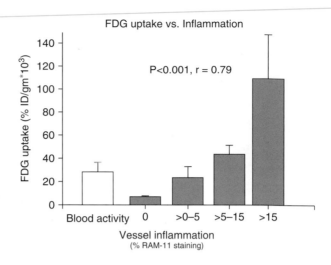

In an attempt to potentially bridge the gaps between currently available imaging techniques and predicting the risk for acute rupture it has been found that fluorine-18 fluorodeoxyglucose (FDG) uptake in plaques is proportional to the degree of inflammation and macrophage density (Figure 7.7).[44] A study of carotid artery plaques in humans by positron emission tomography (PET) co-registered with CTA demonstrated a high uptake of FDG in carotid plaques of symptomatic patients who had carotid endarterectomies (Figures 7.8A and B).[45] However, a more recent in vivo study involving rabbit vasculature evaluated by a fusion

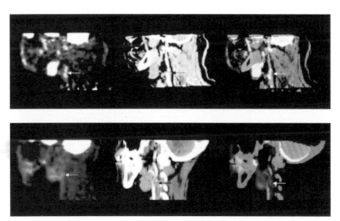

FIGURE 7.8A Top (*left to right*) shows positron emission tomography (PET), contrast computed tomography (CT), and co-registered PET/CT images from a 63-year-old man with history of left-sided hemiparesis. Computed tomography angiogram (CTA) demonstrated stenosis of the proximal right internal carotid artery (*black arrow*). ^{18}FDG uptake at the level of the plaque in shown in the carotid artery (*white arrows*). Bottom (*left to right*) shows low levels of ^{18}FDG uptake in an asymptomatic carotid stenosis. The black arrow highlights the stenosis on the CT angiogram, and the white arrows demonstrate minimal ^{18}FDG accumulation at this site on the ^{18}FDG-PET and co-registered PET/CT images.
From Rudd JH, Warburton EA, Fryer TD, et al. Imaging atherosclerotic plaque inflammation with [18F]-fluorodeoxyglucose positron emission tomography. *Circulation.* 2002; 105:2708–2711.

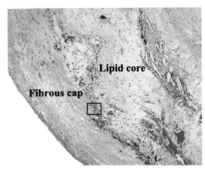

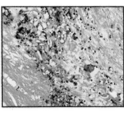

FIGURE 7.8B Tritiated deoxyglucose autoradiography of symptomatic carotid artery plaque (*left panel*). Typical plaque is noted and inset shows silver grains have accumulated within macrophages. Magnification ×10 and ×20.

PET/CT system found that FDG uptake was significantly increased at sites with the greatest inflammation evidenced by high macrophage accumulation.[46] Those were also the sites with the greatest thrombosis and were associated with marked rise in levels of CRP and PAI-1. In the same study, CTA was found to have 90% accuracy in detecting thrombi ≥3 mm in length. Hence, it may be suggested that the combination of FDG-PET scanning co-registered or fused with CTA may potentially be used to identify not only plaques but to differentiate between stable and unstable areas. In combination with serum inflammatory markers, this could potentially be an effective method of detecting early sites of plaque rupture and thrombosis and aid in identifying the vulnerable patient.

REFERENCES

1. Dawber TR, Moore FE Jr, Mann GV, et al. Coronary heart disease in the Framingham Study. *Am J Public Health*, 1957; 47:4–24.
2. Smith SC, Greenland P, Grundy SM. AHA Conference Proceedings: Prevention conference V: Beyond secondary prevention: Identifying the high-risk patient for primary prevention: Executive summary: American Heart Association. *Circulation*. 2000; 101:111–116.
3. Jansson GK. Inflammation, atherosclerosis, and coronary artery disease. *N Engl J Med*. 2005; 352:1685–1695.
4. Lindahl B, Toss H, Siegbahn A, et al. Markers of myocardial damage and inflammation in relation to long-term mortality in unstable coronary artery disease. *N Engl J Med*. 2000; 343:1139–1147.
5. Morrow DA, de Lemos JA. Benchmarks for the assessment of novel cardiovascular biomarkers. *Circulation*. 2007; 115:949–952.
6. Ridker PM. Evaluating novel cardiovascular risk factors: Can we better predict heart attacks? *Ann Intern Med*. 1999; 130:933–937.
7. Ridker PM, Buring JE, Rifai N, et al. Development and validation of improved algorithms for the assessment of global cardiovascular risk in women. *JAMA*. 2007; 297:6:611–619.
8. Liuzzo G, Biasucci LM, Gallimore JR, et al. The prognostic value of C-reactive protein and serum amyloid A protein in severe unstable angina. *N Engl J Med*. 1994; 331:417–424.
9. Ridker PM. Clinical Application of C-reactive protein for cardiovascular disease detection and prevention. *Circulation*. 2003; 107:363–369.
10. Tsimikas S, Willerson JT, Ridker PM. C-reactive protein and other emerging blood biomarkers to optimize risk stratification of vulnerable patients. *J Am Coll Cardiol*. 2006; 47(8); C19–C31.
11. Ridker PM, Rifai N, Rose L, et al. Comparison of C-reactive protein and low-density lipoprotein cholesterol levels in the prediction of fist cardiovascular events. *N Engl J Med*. 2002; 347:1557–1565.
12. Danesh J, Wheeler JG, Hirschfield GM, et al. Reactive Protein and Other Circulating Markers of Inflammation in the Prediction of Coronary Heart Disease. *N Engl J Med*. 2004; 350:14:1387–1397.
13. Hankey GJ, Eikelboom JW. Homocysteine and vascular disease. *Lancet*. 1999; 354:407–413.
14. Knekt P, Reunanen A, Alfthan G, et al. Hyperhomocystinemia: A risk factor of a consequence of coronary heart disease. *Arch Intern Med*. 2001; 161:1589–1594.
15. Danesh J, Collins R, Peto R, et al. Haematocrit, viscosity, erythrocyte sedimentation rate: meta-analyses of prospective studies of coronary heart disease. *Eur Heart J*. 2000; 21(7); 515–520.
16. Wilhelmsen L, Svärdsudd K, Korsan-Bengtsen K, et al. Fibrinogen as a risk factor for stroke and myocardial infarction. *N Engl J Med*. 1984; 311:501–505.
17. Biasucci LM, Vitelli A, Liuzzo G, et al. Elevated levels of interleukin-6 in unstable angina. *Circulation*. 1996; 94:874–877.

18. Yudkin JS, Kumari M, Humphries SE, et al. Inflammation, obesity, stress and coronary heart disease: Is interleukin-6 the link? *Atherosclerosis.* 2000; 148(2):209–214.
19. Harris TB, Ferrucci L, Tracy RP, et al. Associations of elevated interleukin-6 and C-reactive protein levels with mortality in the elderly. *Am J Med.* 1999; 106:506–512.
20. Ridker PM, Rifai N, Stampfer MJ, et al. Plasma concentration of interleukin-6 and the risk of future myocardial infarction among apparently healthy men. *Circulation.* 2000; 101:1767–1772.
21. Vaughan DE. PAI-1 and atherothrombosis. *J Thromb Haemost.* 2005; 3:1879–1883.
22. Vaughan DE, Declerck PJ, Van Houtte E, et al. Reactivated recombinant plasminogen activator inhibitor (PAI-1) effectively prevents thombolysis in vivo. *J Thromb Haemost.* 1992; 68(1):60–63.
23. Eren M, Painter CA, AAtkinson JB, et al. Age-dependent spontaneous coronary arterial thrombosis in transgenic mice that express a stable form of human plasminogen activator inhibitor-1. *Circulation.* 2002; 160:491–496.
24. Sharir T, Germano G, Kang X, et al. Prediction of myocardial infarction versus cardiac death by gated myocardial perfusion SPECT: Risk stratification by the amount of stress-induced ischemia and the poststress ejection fraction. *J Nucl Med.* 2001; 42:831–837.
25. Brown KA. Prognostic value of myocardial perfusion imaging: State of the art and new developments. *J Nucl Cardiol.* 1996; 3:516–537.
26. Hachamovitch R, Berman DS, Kiat, et al. Exercise myocardial perfusion SPECT in patients with known coronary artery disease: Incremental prognostic value and use in risk stratification. *Circulation.* 1996; 93:905–914.
27. Abidov A, Baxx J, Hayes SW, et al. Transient ischemic dilation ratio of the left ventricle is a significant predictor of future cardiac events in patients with otherwise normal myocardial perfusion SPECT. *J Am Coll Cardiol.* 2003; 42:1818–1825.
28. Abidov A, Rozanski A, Hachamovitch R, et al. Prognostic significance of dyspnea in patients referred for cardiac stress testing. *N Engl J Med.* 2005; 353:1889–1898.
29. Morise AP, Jalisi F. Evaluation of pretest and exercise test scores to assess all-cause mortality in unselected patients presenting for exercise testing with symptoms of suspected coronary artery disease. *J Am Coll Cardiol.* 2003; 42:842–850.
30. Arad Y, Goodman KJ, Roth M, et al. Coronary calcification, coronary disease risk factors, C-reactive protein, and atherosclerotic cardiovascular disease events. *J Am Coll Cardiol.* 2005; 46:158–165.
31. Raff GL, Gallagher MJ, O'Neill WW, et al. Diagnostic accuracy of noninvasive coronary angiography using 64-slice spiral computed tomography. *J Am Coll Cardiol.* 2005; 46:552–557.
32. Budoff MJ, Georgiou D, Brody A, et al. Ultrafast computed tomography as a diagnostic modality in the detection of coronary artery disease. *Circulation.* 1996; 93:898–904.
33. van der Wal AC, Becker AE, van der Loos CM, Das PK. Site of intimal rupture or erosion of thrombosed coronary atherosclerotic plaques is characterized by an inflammatory process irrespective of the dominant plaque morphology. *Circulation.* 1994; 89:36–44.
34. Boden WE, O'Rourke RA, Teo KK, et al. Optimal medical therapy with or without PCI for stable coronary disease. *N Engl J Med.* 2007; 356:1503–1516.
35. Loree HM, Kamm RD, Stringfellow RG, Lee RT. Effects of fibrous cap thickness on peak circumferential stress in model atherosclerotic vessels. *Circ Res.* 1992; 71:850–858.
36. Abela GS, Aziz K. Cholesterol crystals rupture biological membranes and human plaques during acute cardiovascular events: A novel insight into plaque rupture by scanning electron microscopy. *Scanning.* 2006; 28:1–10.
37. Fuster V, Lewis A. Conner Memorial Lecture: mechanisms leading to myocardial infarction-insights from studies of vascular biology. *Circulation.* 1994; 90:2126–2146.
38. Libby P. Current concepts of the pathogenesis of the acute coronary syndromes. *Circulation.* 2001; 104:365–372.
39. Kolodgie FD, Burke AP, Farb A, et al. The thin cap fibroatheroma: A type of vulnerable plaque: The major precursors lesion to acute coronary syndromes. *Curr Opin Cardiol.* 2001; 16:285–292.
40. Ambrose JA, Fuster V. The risk of coronary occlusion is not proportional to the prior severity of coronary stenosis. *Heart.* 1998; 79:3–4.
41. Mollet NR, Cademartiri F, Nieman K, et al. Noninvasive assessment of coronary plaque burden using multislice computed tomography. *Am J Cardiol.* 2005; 95:1165–1169.
42. Ishibasi F, Aziz K, Abela GS, et al. Update on coronary angioscopy: Review of a 20-year experience and potential application for detection of vulnerable plaque. *J Interv Cardiol.* 2006; 19:17–25.
43. Amano T, Matsubara T, Uetani T, et al. Impact of metabolic syndrome on tissue characteristics of angiographically mild to moderate coronary lesions. *J Am Coll Cardiol.* 2007; 49:1149–1156.
44. Tawakol A, Migrino RQ, Hoffmann U, et al. Noninvasive in vivo measurement of vascular inflammation with F-18 fluorodeoxyglucose positron emission tomography. *J Nucl Cardiol.* 2005; 12:294–301.
45. Rudd JH, Warburton EA, Fryer TD, et al. Imaging atherosclerotic plaque inflammation with [18F]-fluorodeoxyglucose positron emission tomography. *Circulation.* 2002; 105:2708–2711.
46. Aziz K, Berger K, Claycombe K, et al. Non-invasive detection and localization of vulnerable plaque and arterial thrombosis using CTA/PET. *Circulation.* 2008; 117:2061–2070.

The Future

Plaque Characterization

As technology continues to advance, more work is being done in the field of plaque characterization. So far all the invasive and noninvasive modalities are geared toward the detection of severely stenotic plaques (equal to or greater than 70% stenosis). However, the majority (about 70%) of acute coronary events occur in lesions with less than 50% stenosis (vulnerable plaques).[1] These vulnerable plaques are characterized by a large lipid core, thin fibrous cap, and high degree of inflammation (large number of macrophages). Some early information about plaque characterization came from studying carotid arteries since they are bigger in size and with fewer motion-related artifacts compared to the heart. Using positron emission tomography (PET) images co-registered with computed tomography (CT) scan images, Rudd et al. reported that atherosclerotic plaque inflammation can be imaged with ^{18}FDG-PET, and that symptomatic, unstable plaques accumulate more ^{18}FDG than asymptomatic lesions.[2] On the other hand, Mitsumori et al. reported that multi-sequence magnetic resonance imaging (MRI) can accurately characterize the in vivo state of the fibrous cap, which supports the use of these noninvasive techniques to prospectively identify vulnerable plaques.[3] Most recently, the authors of this book, using an animal model of plaque rupture and thrombosis, reported the feasibility of using CT angiogram (CTA)/PET scans to quantify the degree of plaque inflammation and to detect small thrombi in arteries similar in size to human coronaries.[4] Recently presented abstracts show the feasibility of using CTA with FDG-PET in the evaluation of inflammation in the aortic root and proximal left main coronary artery.[5]

CT/PET

Over the last few years there have been a lot of trials to combine two modalities of noninvasive imaging such as CT/single photon emission CT/(SPECT) and CT/PET. It appears that the CT/PET combination is gaining more popularity. The main clinical use for these CT/PET machines is noncardiac, where it is used in the diagnosis of tumors. There are many potential cardiac applications of this technology; in addition to plaque characterization described above, CT scans can be used to generate transmission scans for cardiac PET in a short time. Also, it is possible to perform a cardiac PET scan (physiologic study) followed or preceded by coronary CT angiography (anatomical study) in the same setting to give a comprehensive idea about the coronary artery and the physiologic significance of any lesions. The drawback of such an approach is the high radiation dose to the patient.

Summary

In summary, we expect that the future will carry a lot of advances in CTA technology, PET technology, and new tracers that will enable better understanding of plaque vulnerability and hence will give clinicians more information to make treatment decisions. Also, we expect a growing role of incorporating serum inflammatory markers with imaging findings and a growing role of combined CTA/PET technology.

REFERENCES

1. Ambrose JA, Fuster V. The risk of coronary occlusion is not proportional to the prior severity of coronary stenoses. *Heart.* 1998; 79:3–4.
2. Rudd JH, Warburton EA, Fryer TD, et al. Imaging atherosclerotic plaque inflammation with [18F]-fluorodeoxyglucose positron emission tomography. *Circulation.* 2002; 105:2708–2711.
3. Mitsumori LM, Hatsukami TS, Ferguson MS, Kerwin WS, Cai J, Yuan C. In vivo accuracy of multisequence MR imaging for identifying unstable fibrous caps in advanced human carotid plaques. *J Magn Reson Imaging.* 2003; 17:410–420.
4. Aziz K, Berger K, Claycombe K. Noninvasive dectection and localization of vulnerable plaque and arterial thrombosis with computed tomography angiography/positron emission tomography. *Circulation.* 2008;117.
5. Rogers IS, Figueroa AL, Nasir K, et al. Assessment of coronary segment inflammation with combined 18-fluorodeoxyglucose positron emission tomography and 64-slice multidetector computed tomography. *Circulation.* 2007; 116(suppl):II_410.

Important Web Sites

ACC (American College of Cardiology): www.acc.org

AHA (American Heart Association): www.aha.org

ASNC (American Society of Nuclear Cardiology): www.asnc.org

CBNC (Certification Board of Nuclear Cardiology): www.cbnc.org

ICANL (Intersocietal Commission for the Accreditation of Nuclear Medicine Laboratories): http://www.icanl.org/icanl/apply/standards.htm

NRC (US Nuclear Regulatory Commission): www.nrc.gov

SCCT (Society of Cardiovascular Computed Tomography): www.scct.org

COCATS Guidelines for Level 2 Training in Nuclear Cardiology

The information below was obtained from the Certification Board of Nuclear Cardiology (CBNC) website. The reader can obtain further details by visiting www.CBNC.org.

COCATS GUIDELINES (Revised 2006)

AMERICAN COLLEGE OF CARDIOLOGY/AMERICAN SOCIETY OF NUCLEAR CARDIOLOGY COCATS GUIDELINES FOR TRAINING IN NUCLEAR CARDIOLOGY

Overview of Nuclear Cardiology Training

Training in nuclear cardiology at all levels should provide an understanding of the indications for specific nuclear cardiology tests, the safe use of radionuclides, basics of instrumentation and image processing, methods of quality control, image interpretation, integration of risk factors, clinical symptoms and stress testing, and the appropriate application of the resultant diagnostic information for clinical management. Training in nuclear cardiology is best acquired in Accreditation Council for Graduate Medical Education (ACGME)-approved training programs in cardiology, nuclear medicine, or radiology. An exception to this ACGME requirement is didactic and laboratory training in radiation safety and radioisotope handling that may be provided by qualified physicians/scientists in a non-ACGME program when such a program is not available as part of the clinical ACGME training program.

Didactic, clinical case experience and hands-on training hours require documentation in a logbook[a] and having the trainee's name appear on the clinical report or other specific record. The hours need to be monitored and verified by the nuclear cardiology training preceptor.

Specialized Training—Level 2 (Minimum of 4 Months)

Fellows who wish to practice the specialty of nuclear cardiology are required to have at least 4 months of training. This includes a minimum of 700 hours of didactic, clinical study interpretation and hands-on clinical case and radiation safety training in nuclear cardiology. In training programs with a high volume of procedures, clinical experience may be acquired in as short a period as 4 months. In programs with a lower volume of procedures, a total of 6 months of clinical experience will be necessary to achieve Level 2 competency. The additional training required of Level 2 trainees is to enhance clinical skills and to qualify them to become authorized users of radioactive materials in accordance with the regulations of the Nuclear Regulatory Commission (NRC) and/or the Agreement States.

Didactic Program

Lectures and Self-Study. The didactic training should include in-depth details of all aspects of the procedures listed in Table A.1. This program may be scheduled over a 12- to 24-month period concurrent and integrated with other fellowship assignments.

[a]These logbooks are not to be submitted with the CBNC application.

TABLE A.1	Classification of Nuclear Cardiology Procedures

1) Standard nuclear cardiology procedures
   a) Myocardial perfusion imaging
      i) Single photon emission computed tomography (SPECT) with technetium-99m agents and Thallium-201
      ii) Positron emission tomography (PET) with rubidium-82 and nitrogen-13 ammonia
      iii) Planar with technetium-99m agents and Thallium-201
      iv) Electrocardiographic (ECG) gating of perfusion images for assessment of global and regional ventricular function
      v) Imaging protocols
      vi) Stress protocols
3) Exercise stress
4) Pharmacologic stress
   a) Viability assessment including re-injection and delayed imaging of Thallium-201 and metabolic imaging where available
   b) Equilibrium gated blood pool or "first pass" radionuclide angiography at rest and during exercise or pharmacologic stress
   c) Qualitative and quantitative methods of image display and analysis
5) Less commonly used nuclear cardiology procedures
   a) Combined myocardial perfusion imaging with cardiac CT
   b) Metabolic imaging using single photon and/or positron emitting radionuclides
   c) Myocardial infarct imaging
   d) Cardiac shunt studies

Radiation Safety. Classroom and laboratory training need to include extensive review of radiation physics and instrumentation, radiation protection, mathematics pertaining to the use and measurement of radioactivity, chemistry of byproduct material for medical use, radiation biology, and the effects of ionizing radiation and radiopharmaceuticals. There should be a thorough review of regulations dealing with radiation safety for the use of radiopharmaceuticals and ionizing radiation. This experience should total a minimum of 80 hours and be clearly documented.

Interpretation of Clinical Cases

Fellows should participate in the interpretation of all nuclear cardiology imaging data for the 4–6 month training period. It is imperative that the fellows have experience in correlating catheterization or CT angiographic data with radionuclide-derived data in a minimum of 30 patients. A teaching conference in which the fellow presents the clinical material and nuclear cardiology results is an appropriate forum for such an experience. A total of 300 cases should be interpreted under preceptor supervision.

Hands-On Experience

Clinical Cases. Fellows acquiring Level 2 training should have hands-on supervised experience in a minimum of 35 patients: 25 patients with myocardial perfusion imaging and 10 patients with radionuclide angiography. Such experience should include pretest patient evaluation, radiopharmaceutical preparation (including experience with relevant radionuclide generators and CT systems), performance of the study, administration of the dosage, calibration and setup of the gamma camera and CT system, setup of the imaging computer, processing the data for display, interpretation of the studies, and generating clinical reports.

Radiation Safety Work Experience.   This experience should be acquired continuously during training in the clinical environment where radioactive materials are being used and under the supervision of an authorized user who meets the NRC requirements of Part 35.290 or Part 35.290(c)(ii)(G) and 35.390 or the equivalent Agreement State requirements, and must include:

1. Ordering, receiving, and unpacking radioactive materials safely and performing the related radiation surveys
2. Performing quality control procedures on instruments used to determine the activity of dosages, and performing checks for proper operation of survey meters
3. Calculating, measuring, and safely preparing patient or human research subject dosages
4. Using administrative controls to prevent a medical event involving the use of unsealed byproduct material
5. Using procedures to safely contain spilled radioactive material and using proper decontamination procedures
6. Administering dosages of radioactive material to patients or human research subjects
7. Eluting generator systems appropriate for preparation of radioactive drugs for imaging and localization studies, measuring and testing the eluate for radionuclide purity, and processing the eluate with reagent kits to prepare labeled radioactive drugs

Additional Experience

In addition, the training program for Level 2 training must provide experience in computer methods for analysis. This should include perfusion and functional data derived from Thallium or technetium agents, and ejection fraction and regional wall motion measurements from radionuclide angiographic studies.

Note: Page numbers referencing figures are italicized and followed by an "*f*". Page numbers referencing tables are italicized and followed by a "*t*".